Lyme Carditis

Adrian Baranchuk · Rachel Wamboldt ·
Chang Nancy Wang

Editors

Lyme Carditis

From A to Z

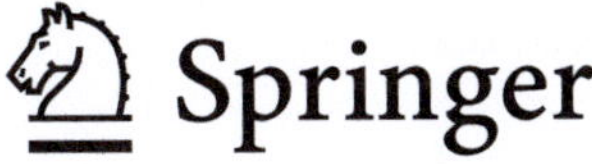

Editors
Adrian Baranchuk
Queen's University
Kingston, ON, Canada

Rachel Wamboldt
Queen's University
Kingston, ON, Canada

Chang Nancy Wang
Queen's University
Kingston, ON, Canada

ISBN 978-3-031-41171-7   ISBN 978-3-031-41169-4   (eBook)
https://doi.org/10.1007/978-3-031-41169-4

This Springer imprint is published by the registered company Springer Nature Switzerland AG
The registered company address is: Gewerbestrasse 11, 6330 Cham, Switzerland

Paper in this product is recyclable.

Foreword

Lyme disease (LD) has become the most important vector-borne disease in the northern hemisphere of the world with Lyme carditis (LC) its most lethal manifestation. Since its initial description in North America in the 1970s, LD has remained an expanding threat to the health of both younger and older populations. As Lyme disease continues its geographic spread in North America, new regions of the USA and Canada have become endemic. Despite its potential for significant morbidity and even mortality, LC remains a largely unresearched topic. As such, clinical LD remains difficult to understand given its diverse manifestations, occurring at different times in this multistage infectious disease.

The purpose of this book is to bring an in-depth focus on the cardiac manifestations of LD. Cardiac involvement is likely underrecognized. Lyme carditis has been particularly challenging given its nonspecific initial manifestations, which can lead to rapid, serious and at times life-threatening involvement of the conduction system in its final stages. Standard definitions of Lyme carditis have historically excluded all conduction abnormalities with the exception of high-grade AV block. These definitions need to be updated in keeping with our current understanding of the diverse conduction abnormalities associated with the infection. This will be explored in further detail in this book as well as potential methods for updating the true prevalence of LC.

Cardiac involvement remains the one lethal manifestations of untreated Lyme disease where prompt diagnosis is imperative to prevent sudden cardiac death and to inform the proper use of pacemakers in the setting of heart block. The Suspicious Index in Lyme Carditis 'SILC' score has an important role in predicting the likelihood that a patient's heart block is caused by LC. As LC is most common in young, active individuals, expansion of the differential diagnosis for AV block is considered in this textbook as well as initial investigative strategies for these individuals. LC in the pediatric population is also discussed by experts in the field.

One of the major highlights of this book is the focus on diagnosis and management of both abnormalities in the conduction system as well as Lyme myocarditis. Emphasis should be placed on early antibiotic therapy for those who are suspected of having LC with admission to hospital for ongoing monitoring. For those with life-threatening conduction abnormalities, temporary pacing should be considered, as conduction abnormalities associated with LC are usually reversible, negating the need for permanent pacemaker implantation. However, for those who have undergone permanent pacemaker implantation, device extraction can be safely arranged if the patient meets the safety outcomes outlined in the included algorithm.

Long-term outcomes of LC treatment are now being explored with follow-up studies showing long-term freedom from conduction abnormalities. Research exploring the topic of late disseminated LC is presented in this textbook, including LC as a potential etiology for idiopathic dilated cardiomyopathy. Potential research opportunities in this important area are summarized in the Into the Future section.

The editors of *Lyme Carditis: From A to Z* have brought together an outstanding team to summarize the most up to date research on the topic of LC. Many of these individuals are leading researchers in this field. We hope you enjoy this comprehensive review of LC.

Baltimore, Maryland, USA   Dr. John Aucott

Contents

Introduction

Adrian Baranchuk, Rachel Wamboldt, and Chang Nancy Wang

Abstract

Lyme disease is an infectious disease transmitted by ticks. One of the earliest sites of dissemination is the tissue of the heart and the cardiovascular system. In this introductory chapter we broadly cover introductory knowledge on the topic, some historical considerations, and a structural outline of the entire book.

Keywords

Lyme disease · Lyme carditis · Atrioventricular block · Myocarditis

1 Introduction

The discovery of *Borrelia burgdorferi* as the cause of Lyme disease (LD) was published in 1982 when the spirochaetal bacteria was isolated from *Ixodes dammini* ticks [1, 2]. Since that time, the geographic prevalence of this tick-vector disease has spread and it is now considered endemic amongst many regions of the northern hemisphere including Canada, the United States, Europe, and Asia [2, 3].

LD is known to affect the skin and joints, but more significantly can manifest within the neurological and cardiovascular (CV) systems. This book will focus on the cardiac manifestations of LD. The incidence of CV involvement in LD has

A. Baranchuk (✉)
Medicine, Cardiac Electrophysiology and Pacing, Kingston General Hospital, Queen's University, Kingston K7L 2V7, Canada
e-mail: barancha@kgh.kari.net

R. Wamboldt · C. N. Wang
Division of Cardiology, Department of Medicine, Queen's University, Kingston, ON, Canada

historically been between 4 and 10% [4], but its prevalence may be underestimated due to the lack of clear cardiac markers of infection (i.e. physical exam and/or surface ECG) in patients with highly suspicious or confirmed LD attending clinical offices or emergency departments [4, 5].

Lyme carditis (LC) is one of the features of early disseminated LD, usually occurring in the first few weeks [2–5]. Patients with LC can present with a myriad of clinical symptoms, which can change rapidly and cause life-threatening illness if not addressed immediately. The cardiac conduction system is the most frequently involved in LC, with nearly 90% of patients presenting with atrioventricular (AV) block [4, 6]. Several reports indicate that conduction abnormalities can fluctuate from first degree AV block (prolongation of the PR interval) to high degree AV block (triggering profound bradycardia) [6, 7]. LC can also lead to disease of the distal conduction system (bundle branch blocks), sinus node, and cause cardiac arrhythmias [6, 7]. Evolution from minor involvement to fatal manifestations may occur within hours, so cardiac monitoring is essential [7]. Additional clinical manifestations during the early disseminated phase include myocarditis, pericarditis, endocarditis and pancarditis. These cases can be severe and some of them may not respond to antibiotics, requiring the evaluation for cardiac transplantation [2, 4].

It is paramount that LC is recognized as a cause of unexpected AV block as it is potentially reversible when treated promptly with guideline-directed antibiotic therapy [9]. The importance of avoiding permanent device implantation and its potentially associated complications in otherwise young and healthy individuals cannot be over-emphasized [10]. The diagnosis and management of LC should be approached using the algorithm highlighted in this book [2, 4]. Each step will be discussed in detail to help guide clinical decision making.

This book will cover many different aspects of LC, however, readers should understand that some questions are still under active investigation. These include ideal diagnostic testing, the association between Lyme carditis and dilated cardiomyopathy, and the role of vaccination to prevent disease in those living within endemic regions. This book aims to share common strategies to help with the early diagnosis and management of LC, including the application of appropriate supportive management and avoidance of unnecessarily invasive treatment.

As science continues to advance in this area, future updates to this book will undoubtedly be required. Ongoing research is imperative to reduce the incidence and impact of LD. It is the joint responsibility of scientists, medical societies, governments, and patient/family led non-governmental organizations to change current legislation to improve LC prevention measures and secure a world with less LD.

References

1. Burgdorfer W, Barbour AG, Hayes SF, Benach JL, et al. Lyme disease—A tick-borne spirochetosis? Science. 1982;216:1317–9.
2. Yeung C, Baranchuk A. Diagnosis and treatment of lyme carditis. J Am Coll Cardiol. 2019;73(6):717–26.

3. Wang C, Yeung C, Enriquez A, Chacko S, Hansom S, Redfearn D, Simpson C, Abdollah H, Baranchuk A. Long-term outcomes in treated lyme carditis. Curr Probl Cardiol. 2021;47(10):100939.
4. Yeung C, Baranchuk A. Systematic approach to the diagnosis and treatment of lyme carditis and high-degree atrioventricular block. Healthcare (Basel). 2018;6(4)pii:E119.
5. Crinion D, Yeung C, Baranchuk A. Lyme carditis atrioventricular block: management strategies. Europace. 2019;21(8):1280–2.
6. Wan D, Blakely C, Branscombe P, Suarez-Fuster L, Glover B, Baranchuk A. Lyme carditis and high-degree atrioventricular block. Am J Cardiol. 2018;26(5):233–9.
7. Gazendam N, Yeung C, Baranchuk A. Lyme carditis presenting as sick sinus syndrome. J Electrocardiol. 2020;59:65–7.
8. Wan D, Baranchuk A. Lyme carditis and atrioventricular block. CMAJ. 2018;190(20):E622.
9. Besant G, Wan D, Yeung C, Blakely C, Branscombe P, Suarez-Fuster L, Redfearn D, Simpson C, Abdollah H, Glover B, Baranchuk A. Suspicious index in lyme carditis (SILC): systematic review and proposed new risk score. Clin Cardiol. 2018;41(12):1611–6.
10. Suarez Fuster L, Gul EE, Baranchuk A. Electrocardiographic progression of acute Lyme disease. Am J Emerg Med. 2017;35(7):1040.e5–e6.

Lyme Diseases Epidemiology: Update 2022

Juan M. Farina and Adrian Baranchuk

Abstract

Lyme disease is mainly present in humid peri-urban zones or rural areas of several countries in North America, Europe, and Asia. Most cases occur in the in the summer months of June and July (within the North hemisphere). The season in which ticks are most active corresponds to the time when people are typically outdoors. People of any age can suffer from Lyme disease, but the normal distribution of this condition is bimodal, with peaks among children and older adults. North America has an estimated incidence of 500,000 cases/year and infections are mostly concentrated in the Northeastern, mid-Atlantic, and upper Midwestern states. In Europe transmission appears to be more frequent in northeastern and central Europe, and in Asia it extends from Western Russia eastward to Japan through Mongolia and China. This chapter will cover the epidemiology for Lyme disease as of 2022.

Keywords

Lyme disease · Lyme carditis · Epidemiology · Endemic regions

J. M. Farina (✉)
Department of Cardiovascular and Thoracic Surgery, Mayo Clinic, Phoenix, AZ, USA
e-mail: juan.farina@gmail.com

A. Baranchuk
Division of Cardiology, Kingston Health Science Centre, Queen's University, Kingston, ON, Canada

1   Introduction

Lyme disease is a tick-borne disease caused by bacterium species of the Borrelia (*B.*) genus [1]. These bacteria are spirochetes, which are motile and spiral shaped. Human illness is characterized by diverse dermatologic, neurologic, rheumatologic, or cardiac abnormalities [1].

Lyme disease is mainly endemic in humid regions of North America, Europe, and Asia (Fig. 1) [2–4]. The disease was named in the 1970s due to an epidemic of arthritis in a small town in eastern Connecticut, and it is now the most common tick-borne disease in North America, where it is essentially caused by *B. burgdorferi* and very rarely, by *B. mayonii* [2–5]. In Europe, at least five species of *B.* (*B. afzelii, B. garinii, B. burgdorferi, B. spielmanii,* and *B. bavariensis*) can cause the disease, leading to a wider variety of possible clinical manifestations than in North America [1]. *B. garinii* and *B. afzelii* are the predominant species in Asia.

Further species (such as *B. bissettii, B. lusitaniae,* and *B. valaisiana*) have been infrequently detected in patients but are not recognized as important pathogens. Interestingly, the genotype of pathogens seems to be the determinant factor causing the diversity of clinical symptoms of Lyme disease [6]. It has been proposed that *B. afzelii* most frequently leads to skin lesions, *B. burgdorferi* is especially arthritogenic, and *B. garinii* is linked to neuroborreliosis.

2   Transmission and Life Cycle

Transmission of Lyme disease occurs after the bite of a tick of the Ixodes (*I.*) complex infected with spirochetes [7]. In the United States of America, the main vectors are *I. scapularis* (also called *blacklegged tick*, or *deer tick*) in the northeastern and upper midwestern regions, and *I. pacificus* in western states [2]. In Europe the main vector of Lyme borrelia is *I. ricinus*, while *I. persulcatus* is the most frequent vector in Asia (Fig. 2) [8]. Even when it has been demonstrated that strains of *B. burgdorferi* can survive under blood banking conditions, no cases of Lyme disease have been linked to blood transfusion yet [9]. There is also no evidence of transmission through sexual contact or breast milk.

The lifecycle of different *I.* tick species generally lasts two to three years, but it can last up to six years depending on climate and host availability. During this time, ticks go through four life stages (egg, larva, nymph, and adult), feeding only once during every active stage and needing a new host at each stage of their life (Fig. 3) [10]. Rarely, some tick species prefer to feed on the same host during all life stages. Ticks normally cycle among small mammals (mice and voles) and birds, but they can also feed from humans by attaching usually to hard-to-see areas such as the groin, armpits, and scalp [7].

In general, an infected tick must be attached to a host for at least 24 h before transmission of Lyme bacteria can occur, and a feeding period of more than 36 h is usually needed for *B.* transmission. This delay could be related to the fact that when an infected tick is feeding, the spirochetes increase in number and undergo

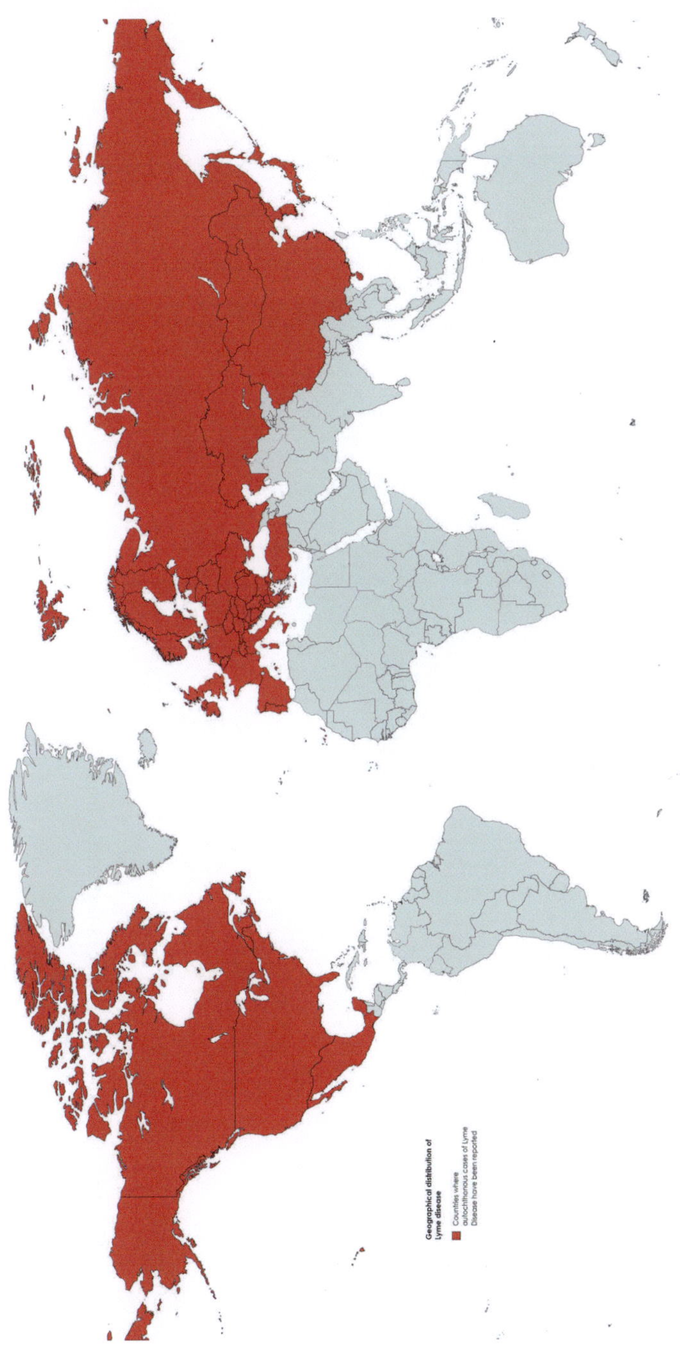

Fig. 1 Global geographical distribution of countries where autochthonous Lyme disease cases have been reported

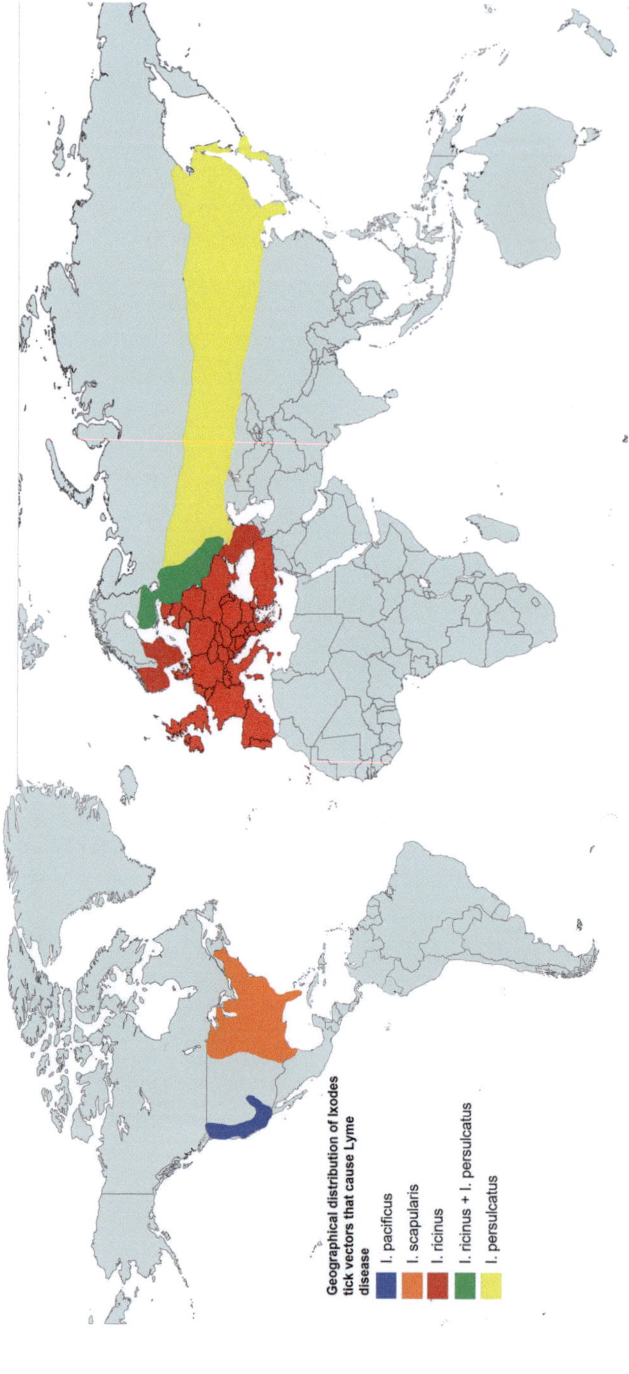

Fig. 2 Worldwide distribution of the Ixodes species that are the main vectors for Lyme disease

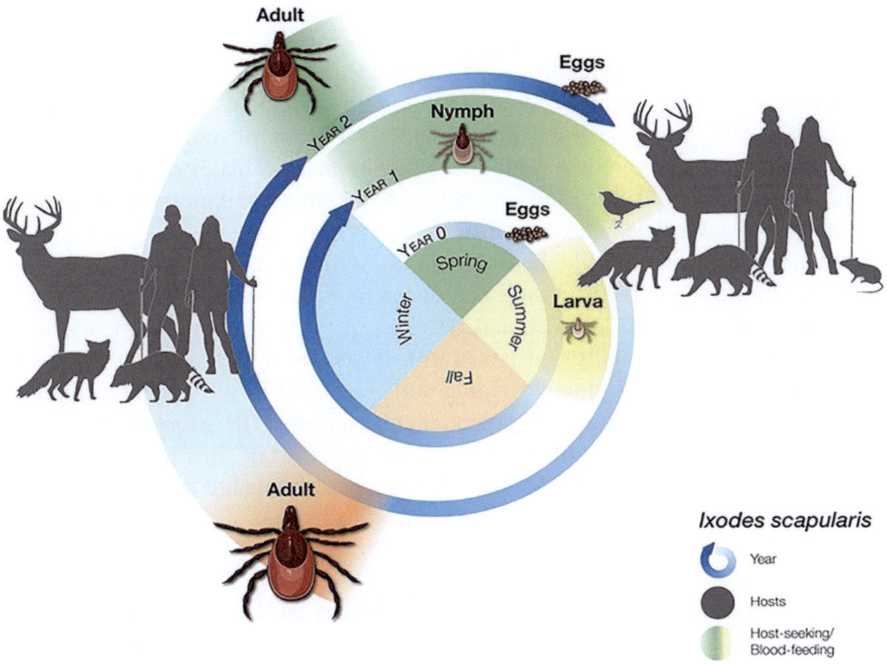

Fig. 3 Life cycle of Ixodes scapularis. *Source* CDC (Centers for Disease Control and Prevention). Reference [2]

phenotypic changes, including the expression of outer surface protein C. This process could take several days but it is critical because it allows them to invade the tick's salivary glands. It is thought that the expression of this surface protein could play an important role in the establishment of infection in mammalian hosts, but the mechanisms are unknown [1]. In contrast, transmission by specific tick species such as *I. ricinus* may occur within 24 h [11].

After feeding for a few days, most ticks will drop off from the host and prepare for the next life stage on or near the soil surface (frequently the tips of grasses and shrub). Deer or cattle are essentials for the maintenance of tick populations because they are one of the few hosts that can feed a large number of adult ticks, but they are not competent reservoirs for spirochetes [2].

Most humans are infected through the bites of nymphs because of their small size (less than 2 mm), relative abundance, and difficulty to be seen. Adult ticks can also transmit Lyme bacteria, but at this stage ticks are much larger and are more likely to be discovered and removed. Ticks can't fly or jump, but many tick species can quickly climb aboard when a host brushes the spot where a tick is waiting. In a proper environment, the ticks take several months to develop into their next developmental stage, and adult females can lay about 2000 eggs [2].

3   Demographics

People of any age can suffer from Lyme disease. However, according mainly to data from the United States of America, the age of patients with this condition is bimodal, with peaks among children under 16 years of age and older adults [2]. Overall, males are affected more often than females. This distribution is likely due to age-related behaviors and interaction with thick habitats (such as outdoor activities) and age-related susceptibilities [12].

Endemic areas are usually humid regions as the *I.* ticks need high relative humidity for survival. Transmission can occur in either peri-urban zones or rural areas used for forestry and recreational activities. A typical habitat for the transmission of Lyme bacteria usually consists of mixed woodland with a layer of decaying vegetation on the ground, thus providing sufficient humidity for the development of ticks, and supporting a range of potential animal hosts [10]. Most cases of Lyme disease occur in the summer months (North hemisphere) of June and July, shortly after the season when ticks are most active and when people are typically outdoors, and the recreational use of tick habitats increases [2].

4   Global Geographical Distribution of Lyme Disease

4.1   North America

In North America, Lyme disease is a highly focal disease, and infections are mostly concentrated in the northeastern, mid-Atlantic, and upper Midwestern states. As shown in Fig. 4, nearly 95% cases in the United States are from 15 states, but the disease continues to spread from these endemic regions to neighboring states [2]. Cases reported from other regions are usually associated with travel to states with higher rates of infection. Exceptions occur in some western states such as Northern California, Oregon, and Washington where infected *I. pacificus* ticks cause some cases of Lyme disease each year.

The prevalence of Lyme Disease in the United States of America has an estimated 476,000 cases annually and is expected to continue to rise annually as climate change increases the range, abundance, and activity of ticks [13]. Indeed, the number of reported cases of Lyme disease more than doubled from 1998 to 2018 [2]. As with other notifiable conditions, not every case of Lyme disease is reported to the public offices and some reported cases may result from other causes. Underreporting is more likely in highly endemic areas, whereas misclassification (overreporting) is more likely in nonendemic regions [3].

As it was previously mentioned, animal studies and clinical observations indicate that I. *scapularis* and I. *pacificus* ticks usually require at least 36 h of attachment to transmit *B. burgdorferi*. Therefore, it is important to highlight in endemic regions in North America the potential preventive role for daily tick checks and showering after potential exposure [2].

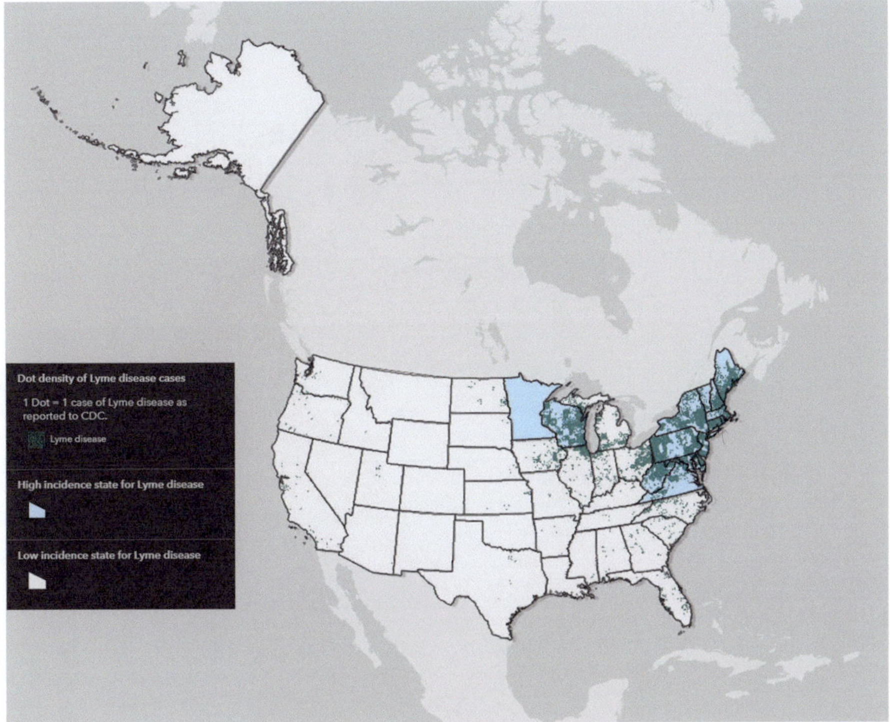

Fig. 4 Incidence of Lyme disease cases per 100,000 in the United States of America. *Source* CDC (Centers for Disease Control and Prevention). Reference [2]

In Canada, the provincial public health units have reported 17,080 human cases of Lyme disease between 2009 and 2022, with an incidence of 3147 new cases in 2021. Geographical distribution follows a similar pattern to the United States of America, as 95% of cases were reported in the states of Ontario, Quebec and Nova Scotia (Fig. 5). Therefore, endemic regions are located in the southeast and center south areas, close to the borders between Canada and the endemic states from the United States of America [14].

4.2   Europe

In Europe, most cases of Lyme disease are transmitted by *I. ricinus*, followed by *I. persulcatus* ticks. *B. afzelii* and *B. garinii* are the genospecies most frequently detected. Interestingly, transmission of *B. afzelii* by *I. ricinus* ticks may occur within 24 h, establishing an important epidemiological difference with the transmission cycle in North America [11]. Tick bites are primarily observed in high season months (from May to September), with the highest peak in June-July.

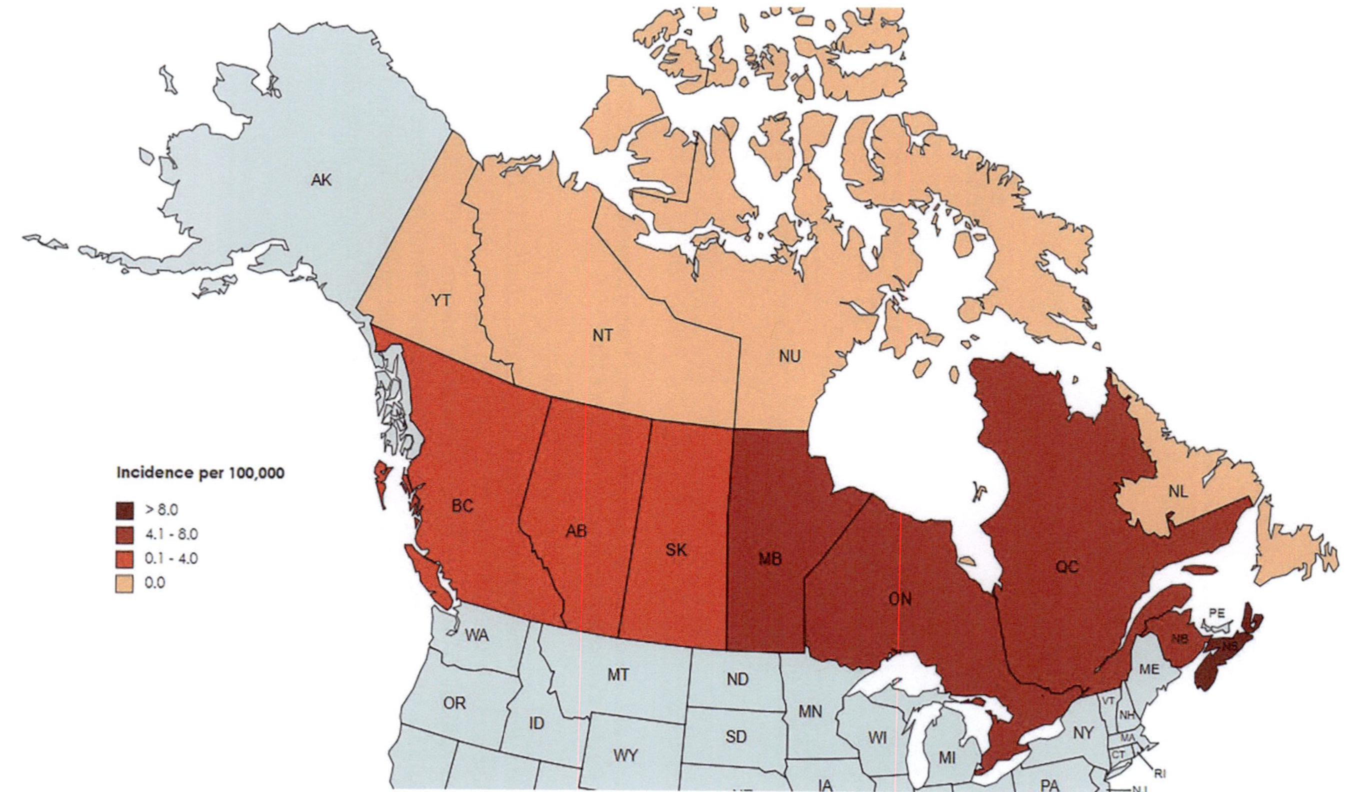

Fig. 5 Incidence of Lyme disease cases per 100,000 in Canada according to the Public Health Agency of Canada, 2019

It is difficult to precisely estimate the incidence of Lyme disease in Europe, because only few countries report this condition as a compulsorily notifiable disease. However, it has been estimated that the number of cases in Europe has raised steadily, and more than 360,000 cases have been reported over the last two decades [15]. In general, transmission appears to be more frequent in northeastern and central Europe and then decreases moving south and westward. Central Europe could be the region with the highest incidence of this infection, as reported by the Czech Republic, Estonia, Lithuania, Slovenia, Austria, Germany, Switzerland, and the Netherlands [16].

Lyme disease is also a continually emerging zoonotic infection in western Europe, approaching endemic proportions in many countries in this region. According to a recent study, the population weighted incidence in western Europe has been estimated to be 22.04/100,000 person-years [17] In this report large differences in country-specific disease burden were found, potentially reflecting the geographical distribution of ticks but also variations in quality and quantity of incidence data obtained and provided from countries. For example, in France, the annual incidence rate was 53/100,000, in northern Italy there were only 1.24 new cases per 1 million residents, and in Lithuania, where this disease is mandatory notifiable, incidence was 99.9 cases per 100,000 population, one of the highest rates on the continent [18].

Further efforts to establish well-conducted and concordant surveillance activities are substantial in the European continent to monitor the disease, especially in current times when tick numbers and activity are increasing [17] As an example of this type of measurements, the European Union has designated neuroborreliosis a notifiable condition and has developed a standard case definition to facilitate comparison across member countries [16, 19].

4.3 Asia

The distribution of *I. persulcatus*, the principal vector in this continent, extends from Western Russia (where it overlaps with *I. ricinus)* eastward to the Pacific Ocean and Japan through Mongolia and China. This *I.* species can transmit *B. afzelii* as well as Asian variants of *B. garinii*. However, human infections appear to be uncommon in some of these countries [20, 21]. The true incidence of Lyme disease in Asian populations is not known, but its distribution appears to be increasing.

In Russia, official records on Lyme disease have been kept since 1990s. Reported incidence in endemic areas generally ranges from 5 to 10 per 100,000 population. However, considerably higher rates are reported in areas northeast of Moscow, in the Urals region, and Western Siberia. In China, *B. burgdorferi* strains have been isolated from rodents and ticks in at least 20 provinces, including northeast, northwest, and southern areas. *B. garinii* and *B. afzelii* are among the most isolated strains in this country, and human illness has been detailed among forestry workers in the northeast region [3].

Both *B. garinii* and *B. afzelii* have been also isolated from patients in Japan; however, the overall incidence in this country is less than 0.1 per 100,000 [3] Most cases occur in northern Japan or, less commonly, from exposures in forested areas in central regions of this country. Enzootic cycles are established in Korea and Taiwan, and *B. garinii* has been isolated in culture from at least one patient from northern Taiwan [3] In Southeast Asia and West Asia, tick infection rates seem to be low and data collection is scarce, so more studies are required to develop more accurate estimates.

5   Risk Factors for Human Infection Associated with Geographical and Environmental Conditions

The risk of human infection with *B.* species is determined by the geographic distribution of vector tick species, local factors, animal hosts, and human behaviors [2]. People at highest risk are those residing or working in endemic areas for Lyme bacteria such as humid forested areas, and have occupations such as forestry workers, gamekeepers, farmers, military personnel, and rangers. Certain hobbies or sports such as orienteering, hunting, picnicking, and gardening also expose individuals more frequently to ticks. Landscaping practices that enhance tick survival (such as failure to clear leaf litter), and deer/cattle density also increase the risk of infection [3].

In the United States of America, the risk for infection is related with different endemic regions. In Northeastern states homes are often situated in heavily tick-infested areas, and exposure could occur primarily in the peri-domestic environment immediately around the houses. In these cases, some measurements can be adapted to help reduce thick populations: clear tall grasses and shrub vegetation around houses; place a 3-feet wide barrier of wood chips between lawns and wooded areas; mow the lawn frequently and keep leaves raked; keep playground equipment away from trees and place them in a sunny location; remove any old furniture, mattresses, or trash from the yard. In the North Central states, areas of highest risk are often less populated, and infection is more often related to travel and recreation [22].

In high endemic areas, some recommendations can be important to prevent tick bites. Before going outdoors, treating clothing and gear with products containing 0.5% permethrin or to use permethrin-treated clothing and gear could help. During outdoors activities, it is important to walk in the center of trails and to avoid wooded and brushy areas with high grass and leaf litter. After returning indoor from potentially infested areas, it is critical to perform a full body check, especially paying attention to hidden areas for ticks and also searching clothes and pets [22].

References

1. Stanek G, Wormser GP, Gray J, Strle F. Lyme borreliosis. Lancet. 2012;379(9814):461–73.
2. CDC. Lyme disease [Webpage]. 2023. Available from: https://www.cdc.gov/lyme/. Accessed on 9 Jan 2023.
3. Mead PS. Epidemiology of Lyme disease. Infect Dis Clin North Am. 2015;29(2):187–210.
4. Sánchez-Vázquez DRMM, Baranchuk A. Lyme carditis: why should Mexico pay attention to this problem? Arch Cardiol Mex. 2018;88:167–70.
5. Steere AC, Malawista SE, Snydman DR, Shope RE, Andiman WA, Ross MR, et al. Lyme arthritis: an epidemic of oligoarticular arthritis in children and adults in three connecticut communities. Arthritis Rheum. 1977;20(1):7–17.
6. Radolf JD, Strle K, Lemieux JE, Strle F. Lyme disease in humans. Curr Issues Mol Biol. 2021;42:333–84.
7. Piesman J, Gern L. Lyme borreliosis in Europe and North America. Parasitology. 2004;129(Suppl):S191–220.
8. Kahl O, Gray JS. The biology of Ixodes ricinus with emphasis on its ecology. Ticks Tick Borne Dis. 2022;14(2):102114.
9. Nadelman RB, Sherer C, Mack L, Pavia CS, Wormser GP. Survival of Borrelia burgdorferi in human blood stored under blood banking conditions. Transfusion. 1990;30(4):298–301.
10. CDC. How ticks spread disease [Webpage]. 2023. Available from: https://www.cdc.gov/ticks/life_cycle_and_hosts.html#:~:text=The%20lifecycle%20of%20Ixodes%20scapularis,larva%2C%20nymph%2C%20and%20adult. Accessed on 9 Jan 2023.
11. Marques AR, Strle F, Wormser GP. Comparison of Lyme disease in the United States and Europe. Emerg Infect Dis. 2021;27(8):2017–24.
12. Kugeler KJ, Mead PS, Schwartz AM, Hinckley AF. Changing trends in age and sex distributions of Lyme disease-United States, 1992–2016. Public Health Rep. 2022;137(4):655–9.
13. Kugeler KJ, Schwartz AM, Delorey MJ, Mead PS, Hinckley AF. Estimating the frequency of Lyme disease diagnoses, United States, 2010–2018. Emerg Infect Dis. 2021;27(2):616–9.
14. Canada PHAO. Lyme disease: surveillance. 2023. Available from: https://www.canada.ca/en/public-health/services/diseases/lyme-disease/surveillance-lyme-disease.html. Accessed on 9 Jan 2023.
15. WHO. Lyme Borreliosis in Europe. 2023. Available from: https://www.euro.who.int/data/assets/pdf_file/0008/246167/Fact-sheet-Lyme-borreliosis-Eng.pdf. Accessed on 9 Jan 2023.
16. van den Wijngaard CC, Hofhuis A, Simoes M, Rood E, van Pelt W, Zeller H, et al. Surveillance perspective on Lyme borreliosis across the European Union and European economic area. Euro Surveill. 2017;22(27).
17. Sykes RA, Makiello P. An estimate of Lyme borreliosis incidence in Western Europedagger. J Public Health (Oxf). 2017;39(1):74–81.
18. Petrulioniene A, Radzisauskiene D, Ambrozaitis A, Caplinskas S, Paulauskas A, Venalis A. Epidemiology of lyme disease in a highly endemic European Zone. Medicina (Kaunas). 2020;56(3).
19. Vandekerckhove O, De Buck E, Van Wijngaerden E. Lyme disease in Western Europe: an emerging problem? A systematic review. Acta Clin Belg. 2021;76(3):244–52.
20. Steere AC. Lyme disease. N Engl J Med. 2001;345(2):115–25.
21. Takano A, Nakao M, Masuzawa T, Takada N, Yano Y, Ishiguro F, et al. Multilocus sequence typing implicates rodents as the main reservoir host of human-pathogenic Borrelia garinii in Japan. J Clin Microbiol. 2011;49(5):2035–9.
22. CDC. Preventing tick bites [Webpage]. 2023. Available from: https://www.cdc.gov/lyme/prev/index.html. Accessed on 9 Jan 2023.

Etiopathogenesis of Lyme Carditis

Oscar Hou In Chou, Kyle Hui, Vanessa Hou Cheng Chou,
Adrian Baranchuk, and Gary Tse

Abstract

The development of Lyme carditis is largely mediated by the direct invasion of the myocardial tissue and the subsequent triggering of pro-inflammatory changes. *Borrelia spp.* modulates the expression of proteins, including outer surface adhesins and complement inhibitor proteins, to facilitate pathogenesis; causing the common manifestations of Lyme carditis including atrioventricular block, other arrhythmias, myocarditis, pericarditis, endocarditis and dilated cardiomyopathy via a plethora of mechanisms.

Keywords

Lyme carditis · Myocardial spirochete invasion · Inflammatory response · Autoimmune response

O. H. I. Chou · K. Hui · V. H. C. Chou · G. Tse (✉)
Heart Failure and Structural Heart Disease Unit, Cardiovascular Analytics Group, China-UK Collaboration, Hong Kong, China
e-mail: garytse86@gmail.com

A. Baranchuk
Division of Cardiology, Queen's University, Kingston, ON, Canada

G. Tse
Kent and Medway Medical School, University of Kent and Canterbury Christ Church, University, Canterbury, UK

School of Nursing and Health Studies, Hong Kong Metropolitan University, Hong Kong, China

© The Author(s), under exclusive license to Springer Nature Switzerland AG 2023   17
A. Baranchuk et al. (eds.), *Lyme Carditis*,
https://doi.org/10.1007/978-3-031-41169-4_3

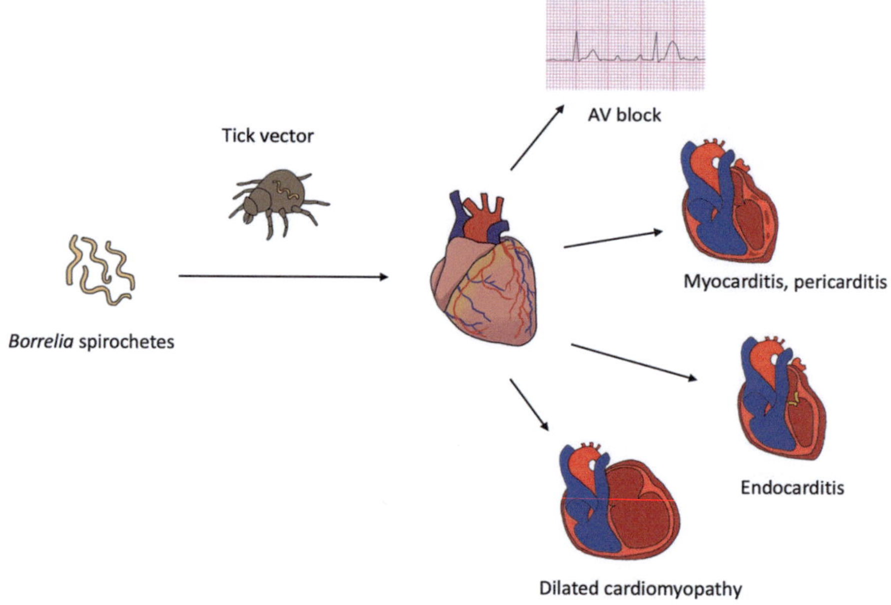

Central illustration

1 Introduction

Lyme disease (LD) is one of the most prevalent tick-borne multi-systemic diseases globally. It is estimated that over 14% of the world's population has suffered from LD, concentrating around Central and Western European as well as Eastern Asian regions [1]. Lyme carditis (LC) occurs when the bacteria enter heart tissues and causes interference with electrical activation and/or propagation, notably at the atrioventricular (AV) node, causing heart block and cardiac injury [2]. Approximately 0.3–4% and 1.5–10% of Lyme infected patients suffer from carditis in Europe and the United States (US), respectively [3]. However, given the prompt use of antibiotics during the early phase of infection, LC is now becoming an increasingly uncommon manifestation. Recent data suggest that the incidence may be at 1% in the US [4].

Lyme carditis is rarely lethal, but sudden cardiac death has been described. One of the most common manifestations of LC is AV block, occurring in up to 90% of cases [5]. AV block typically fluctuates heavily, with the potential of shifting from first-degree to second-degree or complete block and vice versa within minutes. While conduction abnormalities in LC usually involve the AV node, they can occur in other regions of the heart, including the sinoatrial node and bundle branches [6]. In addition to cardiac conduction abnormalities, LC patients may also present with endocarditis, pericarditis, myocarditis or pancarditis [7].

Although the occurrence of carditis is low amongst patients with LD, the incidence of LD is increasing. Rapid recognition of the disease is important as it can be ameliorated by antibiotics and temporary pacing to avoid progression and complications. Permanent pacemaker implantation may be required in severe cases of LC with delayed antibiotic treatment [8]. To avoid this and other complications, understanding the pathogenesis is essential as it will guide clinical decisions made in practice when Lyme carditis does arise.

2   Pathogenesis

2.1   Transmission of Lyme Disease to Human

LD is caused by the *Borrelia spp.*, most commonly *Borrelia burgdorferi*, although it can also be caused by species such as *B. garinii, B. spielmanii,* and *B. afzeii.* In the US, the main causative agent is *Borrelia burgdorferi* and infrequently *Borrelia mayonii.* Meanwhile, in Europe and Asia, Lyme disease is mainly caused by *Borrelia afzelii, Borrelia garinii,* and less commonly *Borrelia burgdorferi* [9]. *Borrelia burgdorferi* is a Gram-negative fastidious microaerophilic spirochete. The spirochetes can invade various tissues in vertebrates, thus infection can manifest in multiple organs around the body [10]. The *Borrelia* genus can be classified by their transmission by hard-bodied or soft-bodied ticks. They can also be classified according to their phylogenetic and comparative genomic analysis. *Borrelia burgdorferi* is further subclassified into different genomospecies, which are associated with respective clinical presentations of LD.

The reservoir for the *Borrelia burgdorferi* includes mammals and some species of birds. For instance, in the US, mammals such as the white-footed mouse (*Peromyscus leucopus*), the western grey squirrel (*Sciurus griseus*), and the eastern grey squirrels (*Sciurus carolinensis*) were suggested as infectious hosts. The bacteria are then transmitted to humans through the Ixodes tick, most commonly by the deer tick *Ixodes scapularis* [11]. The vectors carrying the bacteria vary geographically. While *Ixodes scapularis* and *Ixodes pacificus* are the main transmitters in the US, *Ixodes persulcatus* and *Ixodes ricinus* are the known vectors of Asia and Europe, respectively [12]. The *Borrelia spp.* are capable of surviving in ticks via several mechanisms. For example, the outer surface adhesins OspA and OspB allow *Borrelia burgdorferi* to thrive in the midgut of the ticks [13]. Moreover, the bacteria also express molecules, such as complement inhibitor proteins and TSLPI, to facilitate its dissemination and transmission. Furthermore, the migration of the bacteria to the salivary gland of the tick is regulated by RpoN-RpoS [14].

The ticks transmit the bacteria to humans via their saliva at the location of the bite. The infected ticks generally require 2–3 days of feeding to transmit *Borrelia burgdorferi* to the hosts [15]. The transmission process is influenced by various factors, including the proportion of infected ticks in certain geographical areas, the stage of the life cycle of the ticks, and the environmental exposure to the ticks. Once transmitted, the bacteria can resist the host immune response by modulating the expression of surface proteins. *Borrelia* upregulates complement regulator-acquiring surface proteins to resist complement-mediated elimination and downregulates outer surface protein C to evade the adaptive immune system [16]. During the early disseminated phase of infection, the bacteria can spread via the circulatory and lymphatic systems, thus reaching organs such as the heart and the skin.

2.2   Direct Invasion of Myocardial Tissues

Following the initial tick-borne infection, where the *Borrelia* spirochetes are injected and deposited into the dermis, they proliferate locally, then disseminate to various distant sites within the host. During the early disseminated phase, the accumulating spirochetes can colonise a range of tissues, including cardiac tissues, causing LC. *Borrelia burgdorferi* has shown significant cardiac tissue tropism following dissemination within infected hosts, and have shown to persist within for months to years [14]. In particular, the spirochetes were seen to discriminatorily infiltrate connective tissue at the base of the heart, interventricular septum, and perivascular areas in murine studies [17–19]. These sites of infiltration could thus explain why heart conductive disorders occurs in Lyme carditis.

There is evidence for the necessity of vascular interactions, such as those involving borrelial adhesins, for successful attachment and subsequent colonisation of the spirochetes at secondary infection sites. Specifically, adhesins such as decorin-binding proteins and *p66* have been identified as crucial constituents for cardiac tropism. *Borrelia burgdorferi* expresses a plethora of surface adhesins that can bind with components found within the extracellular matrix of targeted tissues, including glycosaminoglycans (GAG), collagen and decorin. Decorin is upregulated in humans during the remodelling process after myocardial infarction or any myocardium insult [14]. Notably, the adhesin decorin-binding protein A (DbpA) that binds decorin, heparin and dermatan sulphate GAG has been postulated to play a major role in the invasion of cardiac tissues. Animal studies found reduced infectivity and colonisation of the heart with mutant *Borrelia burgdorferi* that lacked *DbpA* compared to wild-type *Borrelia burgdorferi* [16]. However, obtained results vary in the in vivo study between inoculation and tick bites, adding to the complexity of the pathogenic process.

Another adhesion protein of equal significance is *p66*, an integrin-binding protein. It is postulated that not only does *p66* contribute to cardiac tropism, it also promotes the dissemination of spirochetes into the bloodstream [8]. Its expression is inactive within the tick vector, only activating once the tick begins feeding and persisting throughout the mammalian infection, suggesting its importance in pathogenesis [17]. Indeed, an animal study has demonstrated that heart tropism depends on *p66* by comparing infections between *Borrelia burgdorferi* mutants without functional *p66* and wild-type *Borrelia burgdorferi* [18].

Upon infection, *Borrelia burgdorferi* induces changes in the metabolism of the heart, including the mitochondrial function at a cellular level. The large inoculum of the infective agent downregulates mitochondrial components involved in fatty acid metabolism. It also results in compensatory upregulation of proteins in the tricarboxylic acid cycle and respiratory chain processes [19]. This may result in cardiac dysfunction in the heart secondary to mitochondrial dysfunction [20].

Nonetheless, the exact mechanisms of dissemination, invasion and immune evasion of the spirochetes are complex and are yet to be elucidated, and tissue tropism could be strain-dependent [18, 20]. There are allelic variation of genes encoding the bacterial adhesins, which could be the potential explanation for the distinct tissue tropism of different species and strains of Borrelia, leading to different clinical manifestations [21]. It is evident that the adhesion process is not solely dependent on one adhesin, as the deletion of one adhesin is insufficient to dampen the infectivity and tropic effects of *Borrelia burgdorferi*.

2.3   Inflammation and *Borrelia burgdorferi*

As the number of spirochetes identified in the myocardial tissues was discording with the extent of lymphocytic infiltration, it was proposed that the immune response also plays an important role [22]. The increased inflammatory response to bacterial load and the antigen released in the myocardium might be responsible for LC. Meanwhile, the immune processes triggered by molecular mimicry between the bacterial antigen and self-components might also contribute to autoimmune carditis [23]. It was found that the IgM anti-*Borrelia burgdorferi* cross-reacted to molecules that shared homology with the OspA molecule in *Borrelia burgdorferi*. The OspA, in turn, cause polyclonal activation of the B cells and increases the production of the IgM, which reacts with the self-components [24].

3   Conductive Disease and Arrhythmias

LC is closely associated with conduction abnormalities, which can lead to sudden cardiac death in severe cases [4]. The most common abnormality seen in patients with LC is atrioventricular block, present in 90% of cases [25]. AV block typically fluctuates heavily, with the potential of shifting from first-degree to second-degree or complete block and vice versa within minutes. Colonization of the myocardium by *Borrelia burgdorferi* results in an exaggerated immune response and cardiac injury. Research conducted on mice has revealed a correlation between the presence of conduction abnormalities and the inflammatory response triggered by the bacteria [18]. The immune response induced by *Borrelia burgdorferi* leads to a memory-like response in macrophages and causes transcriptional, epigenetic, and metabolic changes in these cells [26]. It has been shown that macrophages are abundant in the distal AV node, with conducting cells interspersed among them

[27]. The resident macrophages express connexin 43 gap junctions to communicate with cardiomyocytes and mediate their normal electrical coupling [27]. As such, the changes caused by *Borrelia burgdorferi* in cardiac resident macrophages, in particular, may alter electrical activity in the heart and result in conduction abnormalities at the AV node [27].

In addition to AV blocks, LC has been associated with sinus pauses, albeit rarely. As of January 2022, only seven case reports have been published [28]. Sinus pauses can be due to spirochete invasion restricted to the atrium, leading to conduction problems only in the SA node [28]. While the cause of sinus node dysfunction in LC remains unclear, there has been postulation that the pauses are a result of SA exit block but not intranodal electrical automaticity as LC is widely recognised to primarily manifest with conduction abnormalities [29]. Bundle branch blocks and intraventricular conduction delay have been in LC patients, making up around 13% of cases [30]. These cases suggest His-Purkinje system involvement by direct spirochete invasion or inflammation.

LC is also associated with other supraventricular arrhythmias, which were mediated by the anti–*Borrelia burgdorferi* antibodies. The antibodies caused cross-reactivity to induce inflammation and atrial fibrosis, which increase the risks of supraventricular arrhythmias [31]. An example of supraventricular arrhythmia is atrial fibrillation (AF). It is extremely rare to see AF in LC patients, with only fewer than 5 cases reported in the English literature as of 2019 [32].

3.1   Lyme Endocarditis

The most recent review of the literature identified only eight reported cases of Lyme endocarditis, all of which occurred in either the US or Europe [33]. Current diagnostic methods of Lyme endocarditis include histopathology, culture, and PCR of heart valves tissue samples. In four out of the eight cases, universal 16S ribosomal ribonucleic acid (rRNA) PCR and sequencing were successful in identifying the presence of *Borrelia* [33].

Due to the rarity of Lyme endocarditis, the exact pathogenesis of the condition is largely unknown. Despite so, it should follow the three critical steps involved in infective endocarditis: preparation of the cardiac valve for bacterial attachment, attachment of circulating bacteria to the valvular surface, and survival of the bacteria along with the propagation of infected vegetation [34].

The endothelium of the heart and valves are normally resistant to bacterial and fungal infections. As such, two models of adherence could be applied to Lyme endocarditis. The first model is the 'damaged induced' pathway, in which previous endocardial injury leads to a deposition of platelets and fibrin that allow the *Borrelia* bacteria to be trapped in. Another model, which is the direct infection of heart valves, could also be possible. This typically happens only if organisms have high virulence. *Staphylococcus aureus*, for instance, is believed to interact with extracellular matrix binding proteins such as von Willebrand factor as a means of internalizing into the endothelial cell [35]. *Borrelia burgdoferi* similarly has the ability to adhere to and bypass endothelial barriers under vascular shear stress. Instead of targeting insoluble matrix Fn deposited on endothelial surfaces, the bacteria recruit and induces polymerization of soluble plasma Fn (pFn), which is normally non-adhesive. Yet, under physiological shear stress, the polymerised pFn form mechanically loaded adhesion complexes that facilitate interactions with endothelial cells via a 'catch-bond mechanism' [36]. After successful adherence to the valvular surface, the bacteria can modulate the physical forces and immunity of endothelial cells to travel through their monolayers, allowing growth and propagation [37].

4   Myocarditis and Pericarditis

The myocardium and pericardium can be affected in LC, either independently or both sites concurrently. Most cases are self-limiting, although there have been a few cases which resulted in mortality, largely in immunocompromised individuals [38–40]. The *Borrelia* spirochetes are known to cause transmural inflammation within the heart, likely through direct invasion and subsequent immune modulation processes described above. Myopericardial involvement in LC has been shown in the murine study by Armstrong et al. [18]. Similarly, in an autopsy report of fatal cases of LC, spirochetes infiltrates were identified in the epicardium and myocardium [38]. Additionally, increased interstitial collagen deposition was found within these infiltrates. This not only highlights the spirochetes' gravitation towards extracellular matrix-like environments, but also indicating their ability to alter the composition of the tissue they reside in, which could explain the colonisation of the myopericardial tissues.

The *Borrelia* spp. is documented to be a potent immunomodulator. This extracellular pathogen is unable to release exotoxins or endotoxins [41]. However, the spirochetes was shown influence the expression of major histocompatibility complex, leading to suppression of the local immune response and evading the host immune surveillance [42]. In the autopsy report, a predominance of lymphocytic cells is found in the infiltrate, which is similar in composition to that in viral myocarditis [38]. In a mouse model of viral myocarditis, humoral and cellular immune responses mainly consisting of macrophages and T-lymphocytes were initiated, eliminating the infectious agent [43]. However, inflammation persisted in the heart for longer in susceptible mouse strains, likely due to secondary autoimmune reactions following infection, progressing into chronic infection [44]. *Borrelia* infections could potentially result in myocarditis and pericarditis in a similar fashion. Myocarditis and pericarditis tend to occur much later than the initial infection [45]. The spirochetes are likely to be able to persist within the myocardium due to the changes induced to the macrophages, then subsequently generate pathogenic cardiac autoantibodies directed against the myocardial proteins.

5   Dilated Cardiomyopathy

A possible long-term consequence of untreated or poorly treated LD is dilated cardiomyopathy (DCM). This topic will be discussed further in Chap. 14.

While the pathophysiological mechanisms behind *B. burgdorferi*-associated DCM are not fully understood, three mechanisms have been proposed: direct invasion of myocardial tissue, maladaptive immune response, and auto-immune responses that lead to exaggerated inflammation [46]. Existing literature is conflicting, and thus it is currently unclear whether *Borrelia* is the cause of DCM, or whether the proceeding inflammatory processes is attributable.

Borrelia burgdorferi defends itself against the host immune system and continues to thrive within cardiac tissues. The spirochete may be able to do so by interfering with all three activation pathways of the complement cascade, through various modalities such as manipulation of its surface proteins and adhesins, and recruitment of certain proteins [47–49]. The inactivation of the complement system reduces continued antigen presentation and thus hyper-affinity maturation, decreasing the capacity of the host to generate effective antibodies against *Borrelia burgdorferi* [50]. The persistence of *Borrelia* in the myocardium can cause chronic inflammation, in turn leading to DCM [51]. Several studies found improving cardiac function and remodelling following the use of antibiotic therapy in patients with suspected *Borrelia*-induced DCM, suggesting that Borrelia may play a direct role in the disease process [46].

However, *Borrelia burgdorferi* may only be present in the myocardium for a temporary period before inducing chronic inflammation that ultimately result in the development of inflammatory DCM [18]. Autoimmunity has also been implicated in the pathogenic progression. Individuals diagnosed with autoimmune diseases, such as Crohn's disease, autoimmune thyroiditis, and psoriasis, have a higher occurrence of *Borrelia burgdorferi*-associated DCM [52]. It is uncertain whether Lyme disease triggers these autoimmune conditions or mimics them, or vice versa. Autoimmune responses have been highly associated with cardiac damage, due to chronic upregulation of inflammatory factors [53]. It is possible that cross-reactive IgM antibodies can react with cardiac tissue with consequent injury and functional abnormalities.

6   Conclusion

The *Borrelia spp.* utilise a plethora of mechanisms to modulate the ticks and human bodies to enhance its dissemination and transmission. *Borrelia spp.* causes LC by direct invasion of the myocardial tissues and triggering and modulating the inflammatory responses.

References

1. Dong Y, Zhou G, Cao W, Xu X, Zhang Y, Ji Z, et al. Global seroprevalence and sociodemographic characteristics of Borrelia burgdorferi sensu lato in human populations: a systematic review and meta-analysis. BMJ Glob Health. 2022;7(6).
2. Rivera OJ, Nookala V. Lyme carditis. Treasure Island (FL): StatPearls; 2022.
3. Scheffold N, Herkommer B, Kandolf R, May AE. Lyme carditis–diagnosis, treatment and prognosis. Dtsch Arztebl Int. 2015;112(12):202–8.
4. Forrester JD, Meiman J, Mullins J, Nelson R, Ertel SH, Cartter M, et al. Notes from the field: update on Lyme carditis, groups at high risk, and frequency of associated sudden cardiac death–United States. MMWR Morb Mortal Wkly Rep. 2014;63(43):982–3.
5. Wan D, Blakely C, Branscombe P, Suarez-Fuster L, Glover B, Baranchuk A. Lyme Carditis and high-degree atrioventricular block. Am J Cardiol. 2018;121(9):1102–4.
6. Schwartz AM, Hinckley AF, Mead PS, Hook SA, Kugeler KJ. Surveillance for Lyme disease—United States, 2008–2015. MMWR Surveill Summ. 2017;66(22):1–12.
7. Yeung C, Baranchuk A. Diagnosis and treatment of Lyme Carditis: JACC review topic of the week. J Am Coll Cardiol. 2019;73(6):717–26.
8. Radesich C, Del Mestre E, Medo K, Vitrella G, Manca P, Chiatto M, et al. Lyme Carditis: from pathophysiology to clinical management. Pathogens. 2022;11(5).
9. Steere AC, Strle F, Wormser GP, Hu LT, Branda JA, Hovius JW, et al. Lyme borreliosis. Nat Rev Dis Primers. 2016;2:16090.
10. Coburn J, Garcia B, Hu LT, Jewett MW, Kraiczy P, Norris SJ, et al. Lyme disease pathogenesis. Curr Issues Mol Biol. 2021;42:473–518.
11. Murray TS, Shapiro ED. Lyme disease. Clin Lab Med. 2010;30(1):311–28.
12. Shapiro ED. Borrelia burgdorferi (Lyme disease). Pediatr Rev. 2014;35(12):500–9.
13. Tilly K, Bestor A, Rosa PA. Functional equivalence of OspA and OspB, but Not OspC, in tick colonization by Borrelia burgdorferi. Infect Immun. 2016;84(5):1565–73.
14. Kurokawa C, Lynn GE, Pedra JHF, Pal U, Narasimhan S, Fikrig E. Interactions between Borrelia burgdorferi and ticks. Nat Rev Microbiol. 2020;18(10):587–600.
15. Piesman J, Mather TN, Sinsky RJ, Spielman A. Duration of tick attachment and Borrelia burgdorferi transmission. J Clin Microbiol. 1987;25(3):557–8.
16. Kraiczy P, Stevenson B. Complement regulator-acquiring surface proteins of Borrelia burgdorferi: structure, function and regulation of gene expression. Ticks Tick Borne Dis. 2013;4(1–2):26–34.
17. Saba S, VanderBrink BA, Perides G, Glickstein LJ, Link MS, Homoud MK, et al. Cardiac conduction abnormalities in a mouse model of Lyme borreliosis. J Interv Card Electrophysiol. 2001;5(2):137–43.
18. Armstrong AL, Barthold SW, Persing DH, Beck DS. Carditis in Lyme disease susceptible and resistant strains of laboratory mice infected with Borrelia burgdorferi. Am J Trop Med Hyg. 1992;47(2):249–58.
19. Barthold SW, Persing DH, Armstrong AL, Peeples RA. Kinetics of Borrelia burgdorferi dissemination and evolution of disease after intradermal inoculation of mice. Am J Pathol. 1991;139(2):263–73.
20. Cerar T, Strle F, Stupica D, Ruzic-Sabljic E, McHugh G, Steere AC, et al. Differences in Genotype, clinical features, and inflammatory potential of Borrelia burgdorferi sensu stricto strains from Europe and the United States. Emerg Infect Dis. 2016;22(5):818–27.
21. Lin YP, Benoit V, Yang X, Martinez-Herranz R, Pal U, Leong JM. Strain-specific variation of the decorin-binding adhesin DbpA influences the tissue tropism of the lyme disease spirochete. PLoS Pathog. 2014;10(7):e1004238.
22. de Koning J, Hoogkamp-Korstanje JA, van der Linde MR, Crijns HJ. Demonstration of spirochetes in cardiac biopsies of patients with Lyme disease. J Infect Dis. 1989;160(1):150–3.
23. Kostić T, Momčilović S, Perišić ZD, Apostolović SR, Cvetković J, Jovanović A, et al. Manifestations of Lyme carditis. Int J Cardiol. 2017;232:24–32.

24. Raveche ES, Schutzer SE, Fernandes H, Bateman H, McCarthy BA, Nickell SP, et al. Evidence of Borrelia autoimmunity-induced component of Lyme carditis and arthritis. J Clin Microbiol. 2005;43(2):850–6.
25. Wan D, Baranchuk A. Lyme carditis and atrioventricular block. CMAJ. 2018;190(20):E622.
26. Barriales D, Martin-Ruiz I, Carreras-Gonzalez A, Montesinos-Robledo M, Azkargorta M, Iloro I, et al. Borrelia burgdorferi infection induces long-term memory-like responses in macrophages with tissue-wide consequences in the heart. PLoS Biol. 2021;19(1):e3001062.
27. Hulsmans M, Clauss S, Xiao L, Aguirre AD, King KR, Hanley A, et al. Macrophages facilitate electrical conduction in the heart. Cell. 2017;169(3):510–22.e20.
28. Buscher A, Doldi F, Eckardt L, Muller P. Lyme carditis manifesting with sinoatrial exit block: a case report. Eur Heart J Case Rep. 2022;6(1):ytac022.
29. Oktay AA, Dibs SR, Friedman H. Sinus pause in association with Lyme carditis. Tex Heart Inst J. 2015;42(3):248–50.
30. Maxwell N, Dryer MM, Baranchuk A, Vinocur JM. Phase 4 block of the right bundle branch suggesting His-Purkinje system involvement in Lyme carditis. HeartRhythm Case Rep. 2021;7(2):112–6.
31. Momčilović S, Jovanović A. Lyme carditis and supraventricular arrhythmias: potential pathophysiological mechanisms. Pol Arch Intern Med. 2022;132(5).
32. Shabbir MA, Saad Shaukat MH, Arshad MH, Sacco J. Lyme carditis presenting as atrial fibrillation in a healthy young male. BMJ Case Rep. 2019;12(6).
33. Nikolic A, Boljevic D, Bojic M, Veljkovic S, Vukovic D, Paglietti B, et al. Lyme endocarditis as an emerging infectious disease: a review of the literature. Front Microbiol. 2020;11:278.
34. Sullam PM, Drake TA, Sande MA. Pathogenesis of endocarditis. Am J Med. 1985;78(6B):110–5.
35. Claes J, Vanassche T, Peetermans M, Liesenborghs L, Vandenbriele C, Vanhoorelbeke K, et al. Adhesion of Staphylococcus aureus to the vessel wall under flow is mediated by von Willebrand factor-binding protein. Blood. 2014;124(10):1669–76.
36. Niddam AF, Ebady R, Bansal A, Koehler A, Hinz B, Moriarty TJ. Plasma fibronectin stabilizes Borrelia burgdorferi-endothelial interactions under vascular shear stress by a catch-bond mechanism. Proc Natl Acad Sci USA. 2017;114(17):E3490–8.
37. Yuste RA, Muenkel M, Axarlis K, Gomez Benito MJ, Reuss A, Blacker G, et al. Borrelia burgdorferi modulates the physical forces and immunity signaling in endothelial cells. iScience. 2022;25(8):104793.
38. Muehlenbachs A, Bollweg BC, Schulz TJ, Forrester JD, DeLeon CM, Molins C, et al. Cardiac tropism of Borrelia burgdorferi: an autopsy study of sudden cardiac death associated with Lyme Carditis. Am J Pathol. 2016;186(5):1195–205.
39. Yoon EC, Vail E, Kleinman G, Lento PA, Li S, Wang G, et al. Lyme disease: a case report of a 17-year-old male with fatal Lyme carditis. Cardiovasc Pathol. 2015;24(5):317–21.
40. Caforio AL, Pankuweit S, Arbustini E, Basso C, Gimeno-Blanes J, Felix SB, et al. Current state of knowledge on aetiology, diagnosis, management, and therapy of myocarditis: a position statement of the European Society of cardiology working group on myocardial and pericardial diseases. Eur Heart J. 2013;34(33):2636–48, 48a–d.
41. Schnarr S, Franz JK, Krause A, Zeidler H. Infection and musculoskeletal conditions: Lyme borreliosis. Best Pract Res Clin Rheumatol. 2006;20(6):1099–118.
42. Singh SK, Girschick HJ. Lyme borreliosis: from infection to autoimmunity. Clin Microbiol Infect. 2004;10(7):598–614.
43. Huber SA, Gauntt CJ, Sakkinen P. Enteroviruses and myocarditis: viral pathogenesis through replication, cytokine induction, and immunopathogenicity. Adv Virus Res. 1998;51:35–80.
44. Klingel K, Hohenadl C, Canu A, Albrecht M, Seemann M, Mall G, et al. Ongoing enterovirus-induced myocarditis is associated with persistent heart muscle infection: quantitative analysis of virus replication, tissue damage, and inflammation. Proc Natl Acad Sci USA. 1992;89(1):314–8.
45. Pilypas AA, Raiseliene G, Valaikiene J. Lyme disease and heart transplantation: presentation of a clinical case and a literature review. Acta Med Litu. 2019;26(3):173–80.

46. Motamed M, Liblik K, Miranda-Arboleda AF, Wamboldt R, Wang CN, Cingolani O, et al. Disseminated Lyme disease and dilated cardiomyopathy: a systematic review. Trends Cardiovasc Med. 2022.
47. Bykowski T, Woodman ME, Cooley AE, Brissette CA, Wallich R, Brade V, et al. Borrelia burgdorferi complement regulator-acquiring surface proteins (BbCRASPs): expression patterns during the mammal-tick infection cycle. Int J Med Microbiol. 2008;298(Suppl 1):249–56.
48. Pietikainen J, Meri T, Blom AM, Meri S. Binding of the complement inhibitor C4b-binding protein to Lyme disease Borreliae. Mol Immunol. 2010;47(6):1299–305.
49. Garcia BL, Zhi H, Wager B, Hook M, Skare JT. Borrelia burgdorferi BBK32 inhibits the classical pathway by blocking activation of the C1 complement complex. PLoS Pathog. 2016;12(1):e1005404.
50. Tracy KE, Baumgarth N. Borrelia burgdorferi manipulates innate and adaptive immunity to establish persistence in rodent reservoir hosts. Front Immunol. 2017;8:116.
51. Yeung C, Mendoza I, Echeverria LE, Baranchuk A. Chagas' cardiomyopathy and Lyme carditis: lessons learned from two infectious diseases affecting the heart. Trends Cardiovasc Med. 2021;31(4):233–9.
52. Kubanek M, Sramko M, Berenova D, Hulinska D, Hrbackova H, Maluskova J, et al. Detection of Borrelia burgdorferi sensu lato in endomyocardial biopsy specimens in individuals with recent-onset dilated cardiomyopathy. Eur J Heart Fail. 2012;14(6):588–96.
53. Pan SY, Tian HM, Zhu Y, Gu WJ, Zou H, Wu XQ, et al. Cardiac damage in autoimmune diseases: target organ involvement that cannot be ignored. Front Immunol. 2022;13:1056400.

Stages of Lyme Disease

John N. Aucott and Alison W. Rebman

Abstract

Untreated Lyme disease (infection with the bacteria *B. burgdorferi* sensu lato) progresses over time through three clinical stages that can present with skin, cardiac, nervous system, and musculoskeletal manifestations. Diagnosing Lyme disease can be challenging, as the initial characteristic skin lesion, erythema migrans, is highly variable, and may present as a single or multiple lesions. Erythema migrans is also not always visible. Patients may initially present with non-specific symptoms such as fever, fatigue, and malaise. All non-erythema migrans manifestations require a positive two-tier serology to confirm the diagnosis. The majority of second stage early disseminated cases are neurologic in nature and may present with any combination of cranial nerve palsy, radiculoneuritis, and meningitis, whereas the majority of late disseminated cases are musculoskeletal in nature. Persistent symptoms may occur after treatment of any stage of Lyme disease, and may be due to a number of potential mechanisms still under study.

Keywords

Lyme disease • Early dissemination • Late dissemination • Serology

J. N. Aucott (✉) · A. W. Rebman
Lyme Disease Research Center, Division of Rheumatology, Department of Medicine,
Johns Hopkins University School of Medicine, Baltimore, MD, USA
e-mail: jaucott2@jhmi.edu

© The Author(s), under exclusive license to Springer Nature Switzerland AG 2023   29
A. Baranchuk et al. (eds.), *Lyme Carditis*,
https://doi.org/10.1007/978-3-031-41169-4_4

1   Introduction

Lyme disease (LD) is an emerging, zoonotic disease driven by complex ecologic interactions between the environment, the tick vector, and human hosts. A worldwide vector borne disease, it is found primarily across large regions of the northern hemisphere in North America and Eurasia. LD is transmitted to humans through the bite of various species of *Ixodes* ticks over the course of a multi-day feeding process [1]. In general, the longer the tick feeds, the higher the risk of transmission. The bacterial agent of LD, *Borrelia burgdorferi* sensu lato *(Bb)*, is a spirochete which is distantly related to *Treponema palladium,* the agent which causes syphilis.

Like syphilis, untreated LD has several clinical phases that reflect the biology of the infection (Fig. 1). Early localized disease (stage 1) occurs at the time of initial inoculation of *Bb* into the skin. Early disseminated disease (stage 2) occurs when *Bb* has disseminated through the blood stream, affecting various organ systems to which it has an affinity. Subsequently, late disseminated disease (stage 3) is typically found months to years later in infected patients. Finally, following appropriate antibiotic treatment, patients with LD may also report a range of posttreatment phenotypes that often significantly affect their health and quality of life. Previous episodes of LD do not confer immunity to subsequent new infections.

Although the specific clinical manifestations which frequently characterize each of these stages have been described for some time, the diagnosis of LD often remains challenging. Patients may present at any stage of the disease, and often do not manifest recognizable signs and symptoms at each of these stages. For example, patients with late stage arthritis often have no recollection of initial signs which would have indicated early, localized infection. In this chapter, we

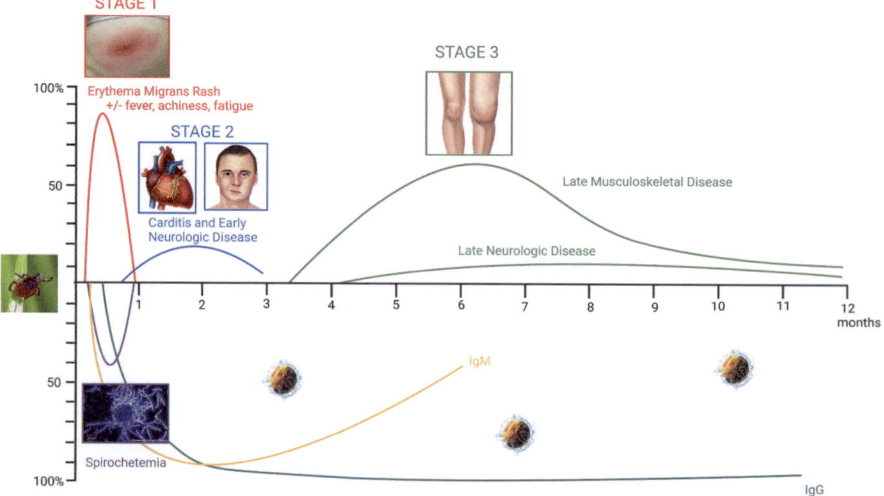

Fig. 1 The natural history of untreated Lyme disease

describe the clinical presentations of each of these stages, along with diagnostic and treatment approaches. We also highlight differences between North American and European LD, which are caused by geographic differences in the infecting *Borrelia* genospecies.

2   Early Localized Lyme Disease (Stage 1)

Although cases of LD can present during any month of the year, tick bites generally follow a seasonally predictable pattern with elevated risk during the late spring, summer, and early fall. Tick bites are not painful, and ticks commonly (but not always) attach to hidden areas of the body, such as the groin, behind the knee, and the abdomen. As a result, a small minority of patients with early disease recall the tick bite or removed a tick [2]. The risk of getting LD after a single tick bite has been difficult to estimate, but is likely < 5% [1]. After transmission of *Bb*, the incubation period of the infection is typically considered to be 7 to 14 days, with a range between 3 and 30 days [3]. There is a small literature describing the use of single-dose doxycycline prophylaxis to prevent LD, which is only appropriate in the first 72 h after tick removal, and is distinct from the longer courses of doxycycline used to treat established LD [4].

2.1   Erythema Migrans Rash

Early or acute localized LD is manifested by a combination of signs and symptoms. The most distinctive of these is the erythema migrans (EM) rash, which occurs at the site of the tick bite and is the primary physical exam sign of LD in the earliest phase of infection before dissemination. Estimates of the percentage of early LD patients with EM vary, but it is generally thought to be present in approximately 80% of cases [1]. EM can either present as a single lesion at the site of the tick bite, or as multiple, disseminated skin lesions (see Sect. 3.1).

Understanding the unique and specific characteristics of EM is crucial to making the early diagnosis of LD. EM lesions emanate from the site of *Bb* inoculation via tick bite, therefore they are most often circular or oval in shape. However, the shape may be altered by specific anatomic contours where the EM is located. For example, EM in the groin often take on oval or elongated shapes, whereas those behind the knee often lose their circular shape when they wrap around to the front of the leg. EM lesions are typically red, blanch with pressure, and may be slightly raised. They may be only minimally pruritic or tender, distinguishing them from other conditions such as bacterial cellulitis. The lesions typically expand over days to weeks, reaching a size greater than 20–30 cm in diameter in some cases. For diagnostic specificity, a cut-off of at least 5 cm in size is expected, although slightly smaller lesions can certainly represent EM in its earliest stage, emphasizing the need for serial measurements in borderline cases. There may be regional lymphadenopathy associated with EM.

Likewise, it is important to appreciate the significant variability that can exist in EM presentation (Fig. 2). While the most distinctive EM pattern is a classic, ring-within-a-ring target or bullseye lesion, central clearing occurs in only approximately 20% of patients [2]. The majority of EM lesions actually lack central clearing and can appear as either uniformly red or reddish-blue. This is often under-appreciated among patients and diagnosing physicians, leading to diagnostic delays. Less commonly (in approximately 8% of patients), EM can present with a vesicular component at the center, which is often confusing for physicians and can lead to misdiagnosis as a spider bite or even shingles. In the natural history of EM, the rash resolves spontaneous over a period of weeks regardless of treatment. Thereafter, this tell-tale manifestation is gone and the opportunity for early diagnosis is more limited.

While characteristic, EM lesions are not pathognomonic for LD. Other insect or arachnid bites may mimic EM, as do certain dermatologic conditions such as

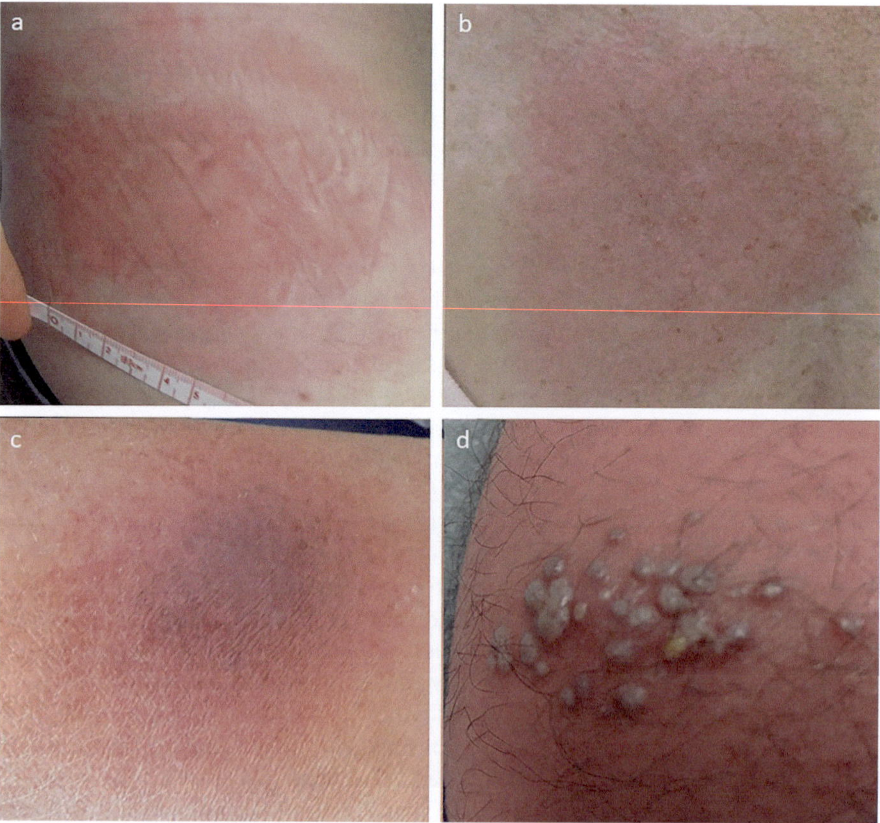

Fig. 2 Examples of variability in erythema Migrans presentation. **a** EM with central clearing and a bullseye pattern. **b** Uniformly red EM. **c** Blue/red EM. **d** Vesicular EM

tinea corporis, although these tend to not expand in size over several days like EM. LD with EM may also be confused with several other tick-borne diseases such as Anaplasmosis or Ehrlichiosis. Finally, an increasingly challenging issue is recognition of an EM-like lesion that is part of a condition transmitted by *Amblyomma americanum* (i.e. lone star) ticks called Southern Tick-Associated Rash Illness (STARI) in the Eastern and Southern US. The pathogen and pathogenesis of this similar tick-transmitted condition is currently unknown, however when it cannot be distinguished from LD it is currently also treated with doxycycline [4].

In Europe, the primary infecting Borrelia genospecies are *B. afzelii* and *B. garinii*. EM caused by these two genospecies have been found to expand slower and patients are less likely than those in the US to present with systemic symptoms, multiple lesions, and/or regional lymphadenopathy [1, 5]. In particular, infection with *B. afzelii*, which does not disseminate as often as *B. burgdorferi* or *B. garinii*, can persist at sites in the skin for month to years, either at the location of the initial tick bite or elsewhere. It can also cause a chronic, later stage skin manifestation called acrodermatitis chronica atrophicans which is noted in Europe but not the US [1].

2.2   Other Acute Symptoms

EM is often accompanied by other non-specific symptoms representative of a stereotypical host response to infection, such as fever, chills, sweats, myalgia (primarily of the neck), fatigue, and malaise. Patients may present initially with either isolated EM, symptoms without EM, or a combination of both EM and symptoms [6]. The diagnosis of LD is significantly more challenging when symptoms present in the absence of EM, as occurs in approximately 20% of patients [1].

Misdiagnosis of LD as SARS-CoV-2 has now been reported, illustrating the difficulty and non-specificity of these "viral infection"-like symptoms which are clearly not specific to LD and overlap with a range of other infectious conditions. Early LD patients without a recognized EM may not only be at higher risk for misdiagnosis, but also for progression to later stages of LD. For example, in a case series of patients with sudden cardiac death the initial presenting features were non-specific symptoms without an obvious cardiac etiology [7]. In the diagnosis of early localized LD, it is important to remember both that LD does not typically cause respiratory symptoms, and that the majority of tick-borne diseases occur in the spring, summer, and early fall.

2.3   Early Laboratory Diagnosis

Th laboratory diagnosis of early LD is challenging. Serologic confirmation using conventional two-tier antibody tests is problematic because of the sero-negative window in the initial weeks of infection before a measurable immune response has developed. Furthermore, convalescent titers in patients who are treated based on the presence of EM, or who are treated empirically for suspicious symptoms, often remain negative in early LD [8]. Commercially-available blood PCR testing may occasionally show bacteremia in the initial weeks of infection, but due to low amounts of circulating *Bb*, sensitivity is quite low. Unfortunately, the gold standard for establishing diagnosis is *Bb* culture of an EM biopsy, which is only available in research settings. When performed in specialized research labs, sensitivity of skin and blood culture and PCR in patients with early LD is high [8]. In addition, approximately 30–50% of patients with EM will have evidence of bloodstream dissemination by PCR [8], setting the stage for later disseminated disease if treatment is not initiated.

In clinical testing, the complete white blood count (CBC) typically does not show leukocytosis or lymphocytosis, and shows normal to mild leukopenia. The presence of significant thrombocytopenia should raise suspicion for anaplasmosis, while significant anemia should prompt consideration of babesiosis. Babesiosis is especially important to consider in patients who have had splenectomy or who are functionally asplenic, as they have a higher risk for severe parasitemia and a higher severity of illness. Mild transaminase elevations in aspartate aminotransferase (AST) and alanine transaminase (ALT) can be also be present in early LD, whereas much higher elevations should suggest the diagnosis of anaplasmosis.

2.4 Asymptomatic Infection

A certain percentage of individuals may have completely asymptomatic infection, or they may not recognize their EM or symptoms as such and recover completely without sequelae. Large sero-epidemiologic studies suggest that the rate of asymptomatic seroconversion may be high, especially in highly endemic regions [1]. It is unknown whether people who have an incidental positive LD serology without symptoms should be treated to prevent later manifestations.

3 Early Disseminated Lyme Disease (Stage 2)

After presenting as a localized skin infection, *Bb* commonly spreads through the blood stream and can cause the following early signs of disseminated infection days to months later.

3.1 Multiple Erythema Migrans Lesions

The most common sign of early dissemination is the presence of multiple EM skin lesions, which are identified in approximately 20% of US patients and 10% of European patients at initial presentation [2]. Lesions distinct from the site of the tick bite represent spread to different areas of the skin during the bacteremic phase and not multiple tick bite inoculations. Disseminated, or multiple, EM can number from 2 to over 20 lesions, and often have a more pleomorphic and atypical appearance. While they usually retain a round shape, they may enlarge and overlap with each other, creating a more complex picture that can easily be misdiagnosed as uticaria, for example. Patients with disseminated EM are more likely to have a positive two-tier serology at the time of presentation [8].

3.2   Neurologic Lyme Disease

Approximately 15% of untreated patients will develop a new, acute neurologic manifestation of disseminated LD on average 4 weeks after initial skin infection [9]. Patients with neurologic disease will present most commonly in the later summer and fall, following the spring and summer seasonal peak of tick transmission. The classic manifestations of active *Bb* nervous system infection include meningitis, cranial nerve palsy (mainly affecting the 7th nerve), and radiculoneuritis (Table 1). Neurologic signs and symptoms may be due to central nervous system, meningeal and/or peripheral nerve or nerve root infection by *Bb*. Additionally, neurologic symptoms such as cognitive difficulties may be due to the impact of systemic *Bb* infection or post-treatment immunologic processes without definitive neurologic involvement, which has been termed Lyme encephalopathy [4].

The clinical diagnosis of neurologic LD begins with a comprehensive evaluation to exclude other causes of the patient's illness. The diagnosis then must be confirmed with a positive two-tier serology. While antibody tests are usually positive during this second stage of infection, IgG seroconversion may be incomplete when the duration of illness is less than 6–8 weeks [8]. In this case, two-tier testing may be falsely negative in some patients and may need to be repeated several weeks later. Patients with cranial nerve palsy or radiculopathy may or may not have concomitant meningitis with abnormalities on cerebrospinal fluid (CSF) analysis. In patients with meningitis, encephalitis, or transverse myelitis, the CSF should show pleocytosis, elevated protein, an elevated IgG index, and oligoclonal bands. Intrathecal production of specific *Bb* antibodies, as measured by an elevated CSF/serum *Bb* antibody ratio, is considered the most specific test for LD of the central nervous system. While very few studies exist, positive intrathecal antibody production seems to be found less frequently in patients with neuroborreliosis in the US than in Europe [5]. PCR of CSF is insensitive and is not useful in making the diagnosis.

B. garinii is a more neurotropic strain of Borrelia that causes disease across Europe but is not present in North America. As a result, neuroborreliosis is likely more common in European compared to North American LD. The classic triad of meningitis, cranial neuritis, and painful radiculoneuritis was first recognized in Europe in the 1920s and is known as Bannwarth syndrome. Rarer manifestations of neuroborreliosis include transverse myelitis, encephalitis, plexopathy, and stroke-like presentations, which are also more common in European LD.

Table 1 Stage 2 and Stage 3 neurologic manifestations attributed to on-going infection with B. burgdorferi[a]

Stage 2 manifestation	Clinical presentation	Neurologic testing
Cranial neuritis	7th nerve (facial palsy) is the most common	Lumbar puncture, if clinical suspicion for meningitis
Meningitis	Headache and neck stiffness are common. Isolated or in combination with CN or radiculoneuritis	Lumbar puncture
Radiculoneuritis	Pain greater than weakness in a dermatomal distribution	Spinal cord MRI if needed to evaluate for mechanical nerve root impingement or myelitis EMG/NCS to document nerve root and/or nerve involvement
Plexopathy	Sensory symptoms and muscle weakness	MRI and EMG/NCS
Encephalomyelitis	Central nervous system symptoms, cerebellar, or spinal cord	MRI of brain and/or spinal cord. Lumbar puncture
Stage 3 manifestation	Clinical presentation	Neurologic testing
Peripheral neuropathy	Sensory polyneuropathy	EMG/NCS
Confluent mononeuritis multiplex	Multiple nerve involvement with mononeuritis multiplex	EMG/NCS
Encephalitis	Cognitive symptoms	Brain MRI and lumbar puncture showing signs of CNS infection

[a] Neurologic symptoms may also result from encephalopathy due to immunologic phenomenon associated with systemic infection not involving the central or peripheral nervous system directly, or after treatment of active infection, as is seen in post-treatment Lyme disease

3.2.1 Cranial Nerve Disease

Cranial nerve palsy is a common manifestation of neurologic LD, particularly in the US [5]. While any cranial nerve can be involved, the facial (7th) nerve is by far the most commonly affected, followed by the oculomotor (3rd) and occasionally the vestibulocochlear (8th) or trigeminal (5th) nerves. It is estimated that LD may account for 25% of facial nerve palsies in endemic regions of the US [10]. Facial nerve palsy due to LD should be suspected over idiopathic Bell's Palsy in bilateral cases, particularly when the onset is during late summer or early fall, and when there are additional systemic symptoms present, such as headache. In one recent case series of patients with facial nerve palsy, 70% had concurrent symptoms such as fatigue, headache, fever, chills, stiff neck, and arthralgias [11]. Occasionally, EM may still be present or there may be a history of a preceding tick bite or rash suggestive of EM. Idiopathic facial nerve palsy is rare among children; therefore, LD should be strongly considered among children presenting with facial palsy who live in or who have visited endemic areas.

Evaluation of facial nerve palsy due to LD should include two-tier serology, although some patients may have non-diagnostic levels of IgG antibodies and will therefore be sero-negative on two-tier testing. Patients may or may not have central nervous system involvement with abnormalities on CSF analysis. In adults, facial nerve palsy occurs in combination with meningitis in approximately 33% of cases [12]. Therefore, particularly in the presence of meningismus or severe headache, patients with facial palsy should be clinically assessed for the possibility of meningitis [13]. The decision to perform lumbar puncture under these circumstances is an area of on-going investigation, largely resulting from continued debate as to whether IV antibiotic treatment is required for Lyme meningitis. In the European setting, studies suggest that oral doxycycline may be sufficient for treatment of LD facial palsy even in the presence of co-existing meningitis [4]. Randomized clinical trials evaluating the use of oral doxycycline for Lyme meningitis have not been performed in the US, and European studies may not be generalizable to the US [4]. While corticosteroid treatments are often used for LD facial palsy, they are of unknown efficacy and safety in this setting [14].

3.2.2 Meningitis

Lyme meningitis may accompany evidence of other cranial or peripheral nerve involvement, or it may appear acutely or sub-acutely as the only manifestation of stage 2 neurologic infection. Symptomatic lymphocytic/monocytic meningitis due to LD is similar in appearance to viral meningitis, with headache, fever, photosensitivity, and neck stiffness. Headache is the most common symptom, with the fluctuating pain ranging from mild to disabling. However, while headache, neck pain and neck stiffness may suggest nervous system involvement due to LD, they are not specific and occur in many LD patients without evidence of meningitis on lumbar puncture. The symptoms of meningitis may continue for weeks to months if not treated.

Due to the non-specificity of the symptoms, it can be difficult to ascertain whether meningitis is present in a patient acutely ill with LD. In one European study of adults with EM and suspected meningitis, only 19% were found to have CSF pleocytosis [15]. These patients more often reported radicular pain, meningeal signs, and larger or multiple EM, however they did not report more severe headache, neck pain, fatigue, or memory/concentration symptoms. As the presence of meningitis has therapeutic implications, it is important to consider lumbar puncture and CSF analysis in patients with a clinical suspicion for meningitis. In meningitis due to LD, CSF pleocytosis with lymphocyte predominance and an elevated CSF protein level will typically be seen. In patients with these abnormalities present, particularly with recent exposure to a LD-endemic region, the diagnosis can be confirmed by two-tier antibody testing, particularly if the illness is greater than 8 weeks' duration. If CSF analysis supports the diagnosis, then consideration of IV ceftriaxone is recommended [4].

Among children, Lyme meningitis may have a slower onset than viral meningitis. Several clinical tools to aid the diagnosis in children have been developed, including the "rule of 7's" where the presence of 7 days or more of headache,

70% mononuclear cells in the CSF and seventh nerve palsy are predictive of Lyme meningitis [13]. Of particular concern in pediatric neurologic LD is the development of elevated intracranial pressure, which can present with prominent headache and cranial nerve palsy with or without meningitis. As a result, evaluation for increased intracranial pressure and papilledema should be of particular concern in pediatric Lyme meningitis. Measurement of the opening CSF pressure should be part of the lumbar puncture, and if elevated, treatment to lower intracranial pressure should be immediately initiated. Complications of intracranial hypertension include transient or permanent impairment of vision, therefore rigorous follow-up with a neurologist and ophthalmologist is important [13].

3.2.3 Encephalomyelitis

Encephalomyelitis is a rare manifestation of disseminated LD in North America, although it is not an uncommon part of the differential diagnosis in referral populations in LD-endemic regions. In the early literature describing LD in North America, case series of encephalitis were reported by several referral centers with presentations including cognitive symptoms, cerebellar ataxia or rarely, stroke-like symptoms [1]. Psychiatric presentations of Lyme encephalitis are well-documented in the literature as well [16]. Transverse myelitis is occasionally seen, and should be considered in patients with a spinal sensory level or in those with unexplained pain, numbness, weakness, or bowel/bladder dysfunction.

Lyme encephalomyelitis is best observed on MRI of the brain and/or spinal cord as areas of contrast enhancement, and on fluid-attenuated inversion recovery (FLAIR) sequences. Non-specific white matter abnormalities frequently observed on MRI are not diagnostic, and have been found to be no more common in the setting of LD than in controls [4]. Patients with neurocognitive symptoms who have normal central nervous system imaging and CSF analysis may have a non-specific encephalopathy associated with LD that is not due to central nervous system infection and does not require IV antibiotics (see Sect. 4.2.2). When parenchymal involvement of the brain or spinal cord due to LD is documented it should be treated using IV over oral antibiotics [4].

3.2.4 Radiculoneuritis

Radiculoneuritis in LD may involve any nerve root, with protean manifestations. The symptoms are usually sensory, but can be motor, as is seen in rare cases of plexopathy. Lyme radiculoneuritis can be confused with mechanical or disc compression syndromes, and occasionally with shingles. When abdominal nerve roots are involved, radiculoneuritis can mimic intra-abdominal process, including appendicitis. In a patient with polyradicular signs and symptoms, electromyography and nerve conduction studies (EMG/NCS) is often helpful where they may document involvement of nerve roots or nerves. LD should be suspected as the cause of the radiculoneuritis in endemic areas when the patient presents in the late spring through autumn months, and does not have an alternative explanation for their symptoms.

3.3   Cardiac Disease

Carditis is the least common but it is also the most lethal form of LD. It appears that males are over-represented in cases of Lyme carditis compared to females. It may present with syncope or sudden death, given the propensity for *Bb* to specifically affect the conduction system within the heart [7]. Many patients with Lyme carditis had a preceding illness with non-specific symptoms and/or an EM that was not recognized as early LD. A more complete discussion of Lyme carditis can be found in subsequent chapters.

3.4   Musculoskeletal Signs and Symptoms

In some patients, musculoskeletal manifestations such as bursitis, tendonitis, and transient arthritis may appear early after dissemination. These symptoms may have a waxing and waning course, they may remit spontaneously, or they may evolve into late Lyme arthritis (see Sect. 4.1) [17].

4   Late Lyme Disease (Stage 3)

After initial bloodstream dissemination of *Bb*, stage 3 disease is identified months to years later in infected patients. Specific manifestations are typically found in the joint and neurologic systems.

4.1   Late Lyme Arthritis

Late Lyme arthritis (LLA) is the classic, most commonly identified stage 3 manifestation of active, untreated *Bb* infection. It was the first manifestation of LD to be identified and characterized in the US in the mid-1970s [1]. It is estimated that approximately 60% of patients with early, untreated LD will progress to develop LLA an average of 6 months later [3]. In the majority of these patients there will be no recollection of a primary skin infection, or there will be a history of a lesion suspicious for EM that remained unrecognized or misdiagnosed.

LLA typically presents as an oligoarthritis with synovitis most often involving the knee in the majority of cases or occasionally other large joints, such as the hip. LLA may be preceded by recurrent, self-limited attacks of joint swelling, tendinitis or bursitis in one or a few locations [17]. Ruptured Baker's cysts are a common complication. LLA rarely involves multiple joints or the small joints (such as the hand) which distinguishes it from rheumatoid arthritis. Synovitis is evidenced by active inflammation and swelling, and fluid can be obtained on arthrocentesis. The joint fluid is inflammatory with a high white blood cell count usually in the range of 10,000 to 25,000 cells/mm [3]. By definition the infection has been present for a lengthy period of time in LLA, therefore patients generally have robust immune responses leading to strongly positive serum antibody tests. PCR testing of the joint fluid is often positive before treatment unlike the low sensitivity of PCR testing in the blood or synovial fluid [17].

While antibiotic treatment of LLA is generally effective, the use of an additional course of oral or IV antibiotics is necessary when there is continued swelling after oral antibiotics [17]. Mild to moderate persistent disease may resolve with time or improve with a repeat course of oral antibiotics. Moderate to severe persistent synovitis should be treated with a single course of IV antibiotics, usually ceftriaxone, and is then considered adequately treated for *Bb* infection. Studies which have examined synovial tissue following synovectomy have not found evidence for visible persistent organisms after IV ceftriaxone. Patients who continue to have symptoms following both oral and IV antibiotics are considered to have post-infectious Lyme arthritis (see Sect. 5.3).

4.2 Late Neurologic Disease

Late neurologic manifestations of LD may occur in patients who were not diagnosed and adequately treated during the initial stages of *Bb* infection. Therefore, they are typically seen in patients 6 months or longer after disease onset. Specific presentations of late neurologic LD include peripheral neuropathy or central nervous system illness, the latter of which remains controversial and is discussed in detail below.

4.2.1 Late Lyme Neuropathy

In early LD clinical reports, neuropathy presenting with distal sensory symptoms and large fiber axonal pattern on EMG/NCS was described by several investigators. North American findings were consistent with an existing, well-documented peripheral neuropathy that occurs in more than half of patients with acrodermatitis chronica atrophicans (ACA), which is a chronic, late stage skin manifestation found in European LD among patients infected with *B. afzelii* [5]. Peripheral neuropathy rarely occurs in children.

In late Lyme neuropathy, CSF findings are usually normal, unlike in acute radiculoneuritis. A positive LD serology, including a positive IgG antibody test suggestive of long-standing infection, is needed to support the diagnosis, as other causes of neuropathy are common in the general population and there is a broad differential diagnosis. A recent opinion piece has questioned whether distal symmetric axonal neuropathy is a common manifestation of late LD [18]. While a positive two-tier test does not prove active nerve infection and may only reflect remote exposure, in a patient with otherwise unexplained neuropathy, treatment can be considered as part of the overall clinical plan. An underlying mononeuritis multiplex which has affected multiple nerves, a so-called "confluent mononeuropathy multiplex", is a more specific finding on EMG thought to best reflect the pathogenesis of late Lyme neuropathy [4].

Although typically seen in patients with post-treatment Lyme disease (PTLD, see Sect. 5.2), small fiber neuropathy may also be common, and can present with patchy sensory symptoms and normal EMG/NCS. A skin biopsy to quantify small fiber changes is required for this diagnosis.

4.2.2 Late Lyme Encephalomyelitis

In the US, late Lyme encephalomyelitis due to active CNS *Bb* infection is a controversial diagnosis with a confusing history. A late Lyme encephalitis primarily involving white matter is more well-established in the European setting, including cases of spastic paraparesis and cognitive impairment [1]. In several early cases series of US patients with LD, central nervous system symptoms lasting months to years were initially described. An infectious etiology was supported by positive serum antibodies and CSF analysis showing inflammation with elevated protein and white blood cell counts. Central nervous system imaging often showed a demyelinating process.

These initial reports appeared to demonstrate CSF abnormalities of parenchymal central nervous system inflammation, however more recent articles have called this conclusion into question, positing that most cases of chronic cognitive symptoms in the context of LD are not due to active infection of the central nervous system, but rather immune mediated phenomenon from infection outside of the nervous system or as part of PTLD (see Sect. 5.2). 'Lyme encephalopathy' has been used to describe subtle, patient-reported cognitive symptoms of diminished concentration, memory and/or cognitive function in the absence of focal central nervous system physical or imaging findings. This constellation of symptoms and findings is almost identical to that seen in PTLD and is not thought to be indicative of active infection with encephalitis [4].

It is important to perform a thorough evaluation of patients presenting with chronic cognitive symptoms in the context of suspected LD, as these symptoms may be present in a variety of neurologic and non-neurologic disorders. When clinical suspicion is high and other causes have been excluded, evaluation should include Lyme disease serology, central nervous system imaging, CSF analysis, and potentially neurocognitive testing, when available. The finding of nonspecific white matter lesions is common in the general population and is not suggestive of Lyme encephalitis in the absence of other supportive findings. Evidence of LD IgG serum antibodies and central nervous system inflammation on CSF analysis should guide the decision for treatment with IV antibiotics. If the CSF and imaging evaluation is completely negative, it is more likely that the patient's symptoms are due to previously treated LD and symptoms of PTLD (see Sect. 5.2).

4.3 Probable Late Lyme Disease

A subset of previously untreated patients may present with a constellation of symptoms (such as fatigue and musculoskeletal pain) but without any of the classic objective physical findings of untreated LD described above. Among these patients, a prior clinical history suspicious for untreated LD and/or a positive IgG serology can help establish a link from current symptoms to prior *Bb* infection [19]. Nonetheless, there is controversy surrounding testing and treatment for patients with non-specific presentations given that symptoms such as fatigue are common in the general population with or without a history of prior LD, and positive serology itself does not necessarily establish active infection, but rather remote exposure. Furthermore, in the presence of co-morbidities, symptoms may be explained by other conditions [20]. The key factor in evaluating these patients is the clinician's assessment of pre-test probability for LD exposure, including high-risk occupational history, or a history of a missed diagnosis of EM in the past. In cases with a high pre-test probability where the patient has not previously been treated for LD, an initial course of antibiotics is a reasonable option. In cases with previous appropriate antibiotic treatment for LD, treatment for PTLD is an option.

5   Post-treatment Outcomes

The prognosis after antibiotic treatment for patients with LD is generally good, with prevention of most new objective signs of ongoing infection, including progression to subsequent disease stages [1]. An exception is the small number of cases that develop early neurologic disease, particularly 7th nerve palsy, in the first few days after doxycycline is initiated for early LD. Despite this favorable prognosis, there are well-documented cases of post-treatment symptoms following what is considered adequate antibiotic treatment of the infection. These post-treatment symptoms can be considered infection-associated chronic illnesses, a category of illnesses which have long been described following a host of viral and bacterial pathogens [21]. While the broadest group of such patients, who may or may not have evidence of prior LD, are often termed to have chronic Lyme disease, there are more defined, research-based patient subsets of this group that can be identified, as described below [22].

5.1   Chronic Lyme Disease

In the current medical literature, chronic Lyme disease (CLD) is viewed as a non-specific term which encompasses a widely heterogenous group of patients who share common but non-specific symptoms such as fatigue, memory issues, and pain that remain unexplained after often extensive testing [23]. The topic of CLD has historically been difficult because of controversy and confusion surrounding its diagnosis, severity, and treatment. Such patients may have no clinical history or laboratory evidence of LD, or they may have suspicious histories but fail to meet specific case definitions for LD or post-treatment Lyme disease (see Sect. 5.2). Similar to the imprecise diagnosis of 'chest pain' for example, where not all patients will end up with a cardiac cause, some patients with CLD may have other distinct diagnoses unrelated to LD that become apparent after further investigation. Other patients may also meet case definitions for clinically similar syndromes such as myalgic encephalomyelitis/chronic fatigue syndrome or fibromyalgia. Among patients with non-specific symptoms, it is challenging to ascribe their illness to LD, in particular given the lack of sensitivity of serology in establishing initial exposure to *Bb* infection. In cases where LD was initially mis-diagnosed or improperly treated, this because especially difficult. The proper classification of these patients awaits improvements in diagnostic testing and a better understanding of the potential shared mechanisms of these symptoms.

5.2   Post-treatment Lyme Disease

Post-treatment Lyme disease (PTLD) represents a specific sub-group of patients with CLD whose symptoms can be more readily linked to a prior history of LD [22]. Among all patients presenting for evaluation of CLD in large referral practices, the proportion who meet criteria for PTLD has varied across studies but is estimated to be approximately 10% [24]. A strict research case definition was proposed by the Infectious Diseases Society of America (IDSA) in 2006 which includes clear prior LD, the absence of specific co-morbidities, the presence of functionally impairing fatigue, widespread pain, and/or cognitive dysfunction, and symptoms of at least 6 months' duration [25]. The non-resolving or recurrent symptoms of PTLD, which commonly include those listed in the IDSA case definition as well as additional sleep, neurologic, visual, and mood-based symptoms, can occur after treatment of all stages of LD.

Patient-reported or so-called 'subjective' symptoms are the key clinical feature of PTLD. While the lack of objective physical findings renders them more difficult to document, patients often report significant symptom burden and impacts on health-related quality of life [22]. It is true that PTLD symptoms are non-specific and are commonly noted in other conditions and in the general population. However, their prevalence and magnitude typically render them more impactful. While many of the symptoms of PTLD can overlap with the initial pre-treatment symptoms of early LD (such as fatigue, pain and cognitive complaints suggestive of encephalopathy), other acute infectious symptoms such as fever are less frequently present. A large registry study in Europe found that patients with a hospital-based LD diagnosis had an increased risk of mental disorders and suicide in subsequent months to years, and psychiatric symptoms may be a common downstream component of PTLD [26].

PTLD may be temporary and resolve with time after treatment as part of the normal recovery from LD infection, or these symptoms have been documented to persist or reoccur for over a decade in some cases [1]. There is no FDA-approved therapy for PTLD, however treatment of associated conditions such as inflammatory arthritis, postural orthostatic tachycardia syndrome (POTS), sleep disruption, and anxiety, is essential. Several treatment trials testing repeated courses of antibiotic therapy have been conducted and have shown some improvement in fatigue but have failed to show a curative benefit [24], however their study designs and conclusions have been debated. It does seem clear that optimal therapy of PTLD has not been developed. This raises the question of whether other downstream disease mechanisms may be involved in maintaining this condition.

Prospective studies conducted in the US have estimated that among early LD patients with EM treated promptly and appropriately, the rate of PTLD is 10–20% [27, 28], depending on the outcome definition applied. In Europe, these rates are reportedly higher among patients with neuroborreliosis and lower among patients with EM. This variability is likely due to differences in the infecting strains [5]. In general, the presence of neurologic symptoms as well as a more severe initial course of LD are considered risk factors for the development of PTLD. Additionally, delays in diagnosis and treatment and non-EM initial presentation of disease have been identified as risk factors as well. Other studies have identified associations between risk of PTLD and female sex, older age, co-morbid medical conditions, and psychological factors such as a higher number of prior stressful life events [24]. Although more research is needed, it appears that PTLD occurs less frequently in children compared to adults.

Several hypotheses exist regarding the pathogenesis of PTLD, including a dysregulated immune response, microbial mechanisms, and neural network alterations (Fig. 3) [22, 24]. Based on in-vitro and animal studies, some have postulated that PTLD is driven by persistent underlying *Bb* infection that was not fully cleared by antibiotic therapy. Alternatively, is it hypothesized that symptoms can be driven by persistent inflammation caused by bacterial antigen in the absence of viable organisms and/or the development of auto-immune processes. The relevance of other tick-borne infections or co-infections, including *B. miyamotoi*, babesiosis, and bartonellosis, has received very little study and their role in PTLD remains unexplored. Finally, there is likely some overlap in the mechanism and maintenance of common symptoms such as fatigue across infection-associated chronic illnesses such as PTLD, ME/CFS and post-acute SARS-COV-2 that awaits future research. This could include changes in the microbiome, autonomic dysregulation, and/or psychosocial factors associated with illness uncertainty and invalidation.

5.3 Post-infectious Lyme Arthritis

Post-infectious Lyme arthritis (PILA), (previously called antibiotic-refractory late Lyme arthritis) represents another subset of more clearly defined patients with symptoms following appropriate treatment for LD. PILA occurs in approximately 10% of cases after what is deemed appropriate antibiotic treatment for late Lyme arthritis, typically several courses of oral antibiotics and often a single course of intravenous ceftriaxone. Despite these treatments, patients continue to have persistent synovitis and joint swelling, typically manifest as oligoarthritis of the knee. Patients with PILA always have a well-documented history of recently treated late Lyme arthritis, and are almost always strongly positive on serologic testing.

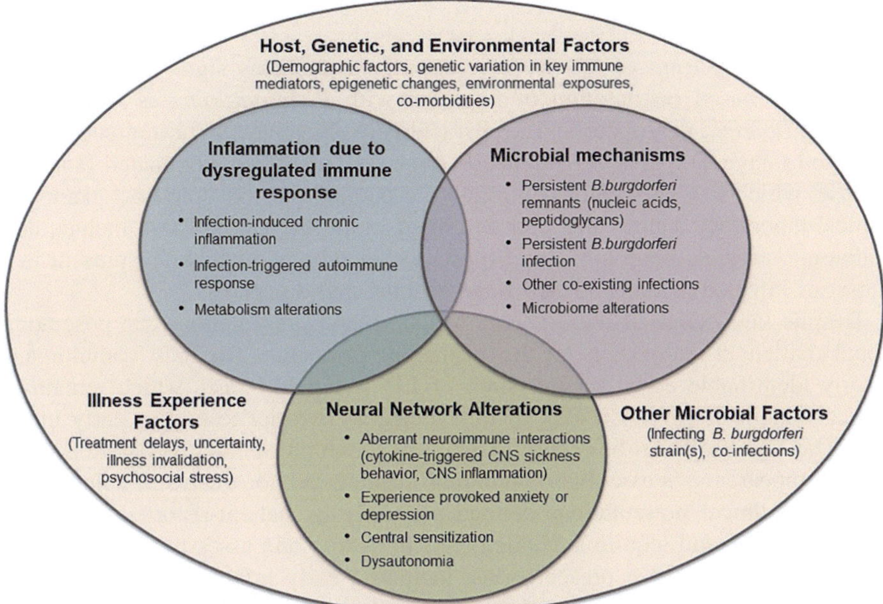

Fig. 3 Hypotheses regarding potential mechanisms of post-treatment Lyme disease. Adapted/updated from Rebman et al. [22]

Bb is not seen in pathology specimens from patients undergoing synovectomy for PILA, and studies examining synovial fluid PCR have concluded that residual *Bb* infection is not the mechanism of on-going joint inflammation. However, other studies have implicated the presence of residual *Bb* peptidoglycan antigens in the pathophysiology of this condition, therefore not excluding a role for ongoing microbial stimulation of persistent inflammation in this condition [17]. Other studies have supported the role of autoimmunity in the pathogenesis of PILD, and a long history of non-controlled treatment studies has shown that following several courses of antibiotics, treatments that focus on immune suppression such as plaquenil, methotrexate, and TNF inhibitors, can be successful [17].

In contrast to the oligoarthritis of PILA, some patients with a prior history of treated LD may present with small joint arthritis in a pattern resembling that seen in psoriatic arthritis, spondyloarthropathy, or rheumatoid arthritis. Often, multiple joints and/or entheses are involved. These inflammatory arthridities occurs more often months to years later in the context of previously treated early LD, rather than late Lyme arthritis. The association of these arthridities with prior LD has not been fully explored however, and LD has not been proven to be a risk factor in these conditions [29].

6 Conclusions

The clinical spectrum of LD is diverse and encompasses signs and symptoms which vary based on duration of infection with *B. burgdorferi* as well as the infecting *Borrelia* genospecies. The characteristic objective manifestations of early localized (stage 1), early disseminated (stage 2), and late disseminated (stage 3) disease, which can be identified through the patient's history, physical exam and clinical laboratory testing, are well-described in the literature. These include dermatologic, cardiac, neurologic, and musculoskeletal signs which are present in a subset of infected patients at each stage of untreated disease.

Despite knowledge of these classic signs, several presentations can pose additional challenges and pitfalls for the diagnosing physician. The most common and readily identifiable early manifestation of LD is the EM rash, which remains a clinical diagnosis given the risk of false negative two-tier testing in early infection. The EM itself can be highly variable in presentation, and recognition of its diverse appearance is essential to avoiding misdiagnosis or treatment delays. Furthermore, clinical presentations defined primarily by patient-reported symptoms are problematic and require a detailed clinical history and assessment of exposure risk. Patients with these presentations, including early infection without a rash, cases where symptoms precede objective manifestations, and late neurologic disease, would also greatly benefit from scientific advances in testing to aid prompt and accurate diagnosis.

Given the increasing incidence and expanding geography of LD, the cumulative prevalence of patients with post-treatment symptoms is an area of increasing impact and concern. In patients appropriately treated with continued symptoms, two-tier serology is unhelpful in diagnosis or evaluating treatment response. There is a significant unmet need for research to understand the shared underlying mechanisms of PTLD and other infection-associated chronic illnesses, as well as advance therapeutics to address symptom burden in these conditions.

References

1. Steere AC, Strle F, Wormser GP, et al. Lyme borreliosis. Nat Rev Dis Primers. 2016;2:16090. https://doi.org/10.1038/nrdp.2016.90.
2. Tibbles CD, Edlow JA. Does this patient have erythema migrans? JAMA. 2007;297(23):2617–27. https://doi.org/10.1001/jama.297.23.2617.
3. Wormser GP. Early Lyme Disease. N Engl J Med. 2006;354:2794–801. https://doi.org/10.1056/NEJMcp061181.
4. Lantos PM, Rumbaugh J, Bockenstedt LK, et al. Clinical practice guidelines by the infectious diseases society of America (IDSA), American academy of neurology (AAN), and American college of rheumatology (ACR): 2020 guidelines for the prevention, diagnosis and treatment of Lyme disease. Clin Infect Dis. 2021;72(1):1–8. https://doi.org/10.1093/cid/ciab049.
5. Marques AR, Strle F, Wormser GP. Comparison of Lyme disease in the United States and Europe. Emerg Infect Dis. 2021;27(8):2017–24. https://doi.org/10.3201/EID2708.204763.

6. Rebman AW, Yang T, Yoon I, Powell D, Geller SA, Aucott JN. Initial presentation and time to treatment in early Lyme disease. Am J Trop Med Hyg. Published online 6 Feb 2023. https://doi.org/10.4269/AJTMH.22-0437.

7. Centers for Disease Control and Prevention. Three sudden cardiac deaths associated with Lyme carditis—United States, November 2012–July 2013. MMWR Morb Mortal Wkly Rep. 2013;62(49):993–6. http://www.ncbi.nlm.nih.gov/pubmed/24336130.

8. Branda JA, Steere AC. Laboratory diagnosis of Lyme Borreliosis. Clin Microbiol Rev. 2021;34(2):1–45. https://doi.org/10.1128/CMR.00018-19.

9. Marques AR. Lyme Neuroborreliosis. Continuum (Minneap Minn). 2015;21(6 Neuroinfectious Disease):1729–44. https://doi.org/10.1212/con.0000000000000252.

10. Halperin JJ. Neuroborreliosis. Neurol Clin. 2018;36(4):821–30. https://doi.org/10.1016/J.NCL.2018.06.006.

11. Marques A, Okpali G, Liepshutz K, Ortega-Villa AM. Characteristics and outcome of facial nerve palsy from Lyme neuroborreliosis in the United States. Ann Clin Transl Neurol. 2022;9(1):41–9. https://doi.org/10.1002/ACN3.51488.

12. Halperin JJ. Facial nerve palsy associated with Lyme disease. Muscle Nerve. 2003;28(4):516–7. https://doi.org/10.1002/mus.10451.

13. Sood SK. Lyme disease in children. Infect Dis Clin North Am. 2015;29(2):281–94. https://doi.org/10.1016/J.IDC.2015.02.011.

14. Wormser GP, McKenna D, Scavarda C, Karmen C. Outcome of facial palsy from Lyme disease in prospectively followed patients who had received corticosteroids. Diagn Microbiol Infect Dis. 2018;91(4):336–8. https://doi.org/10.1016/j.diagmicrobio.2018.03.016.

15. Ogrinc K, Lotric-Furlan S, Maraspin V, et al. Suspected early Lyme neuroborreliosis in patients with erythema migrans. Clin Infect Dis. 2013;57(4):501–9. https://doi.org/10.1093/cid/cit317.

16. Fallon BA, Nields JA, Burrascano JJ, Liegner K, DelBene D, Liebowitz MR. The neuropsychiatric manifestations of Lyme borreliosis. Psychiatr Q. 1992;63(1):95–117. http://www.ncbi.nlm.nih.gov/pubmed/1438607.

17. Arvikar SL, Steere AC. Lyme arthritis. Infect Dis Clin North Am. 2022;36(3):563–77. https://doi.org/10.1016/J.IDC.2022.03.006.

18. Wormser GP, Strle F, Shapiro ED, Dattwyler RJ, Auwaerter PG. A critical appraisal of the mild axonal peripheral neuropathy of late neurologic Lyme disease. Diagn Microbiol Infect Dis. 2017;87(2):163–7. https://doi.org/10.1016/j.diagmicrobio.2016.11.003.

19. Aucott JN, Seifter A, Rebman AW. Probable late Lyme disease: a variant manifestation of untreated Borrelia burgdorferi infection. BMC Infect Dis. 2012;12:173. https://doi.org/10.1186/1471-2334-12-173.

20. Tugwell P, Dennis DT, Weinstein A, et al. Laboratory evaluation in the diagnosis of Lyme disease. Ann Intern Med. 1997;127(12):1109–1123. http://www.ncbi.nlm.nih.gov/pubmed/9412316.

21. Choutka J, Jansari V, Hornig M, Iwasaki A. Unexplained post-acute infection syndromes. Nat Med. 2022;28(5):911–23. https://doi.org/10.1038/s41591-022-01810-6.

22. Rebman AW, Aucott JN. Post-treatment Lyme disease as a model for persistent symptoms in Lyme disease. Front Med (Lausanne). 2020;7(57). https://doi.org/10.3389/fmed.2020.00057.

23. Feder HM Jr, Johnson BJ, O'Connell S, et al. A critical appraisal of "chronic Lyme disease." N Engl J Med. 2007;357(14):1422–30. https://doi.org/10.1056/NEJMra072023.

24. Marques A. Persistent symptoms after treatment of Lyme disease. Infect Dis Clin North Am. 2022;36(3):621–38. https://doi.org/10.1016/J.IDC.2022.04.004.

25. Wormser GP, Dattwyler RJ, Shapiro ED, et al. The clinical assessment, treatment, and prevention of Lyme disease, human granulocytic anaplasmosis, and babesiosis: clinical practice guidelines by the infectious diseases society of America. Clin Infect Dis. 2006;43(9):1089–134. https://doi.org/10.1086/508667.

26. Fallon BA, Madsen T, Erlangsen A, Benros ME. Lyme borreliosis and associations with mental disorders and suicidal behavior: a nationwide Danish cohort study. Am J Psychiatry. 2021;178(10):921–31. https://doi.org/10.1176/APPI.AJP.2021.20091347/ASSET/IMAGES/LARGE/APPI.AJP.2021.20091347F2.JPEG.

27. Aucott JN, Yang T, Yoon I, Powell D, Geller SA, Rebman AW. Risk of post-treatment Lyme disease in patients with ideally-treated early Lyme disease: a prospective cohort study. Int J Infect Dis. 2022;116:230–7. https://doi.org/10.1016/J.IJID.2022.01.033.
28. Wormser GP, McKenna D, Karmen CL, et al. Prospective evaluation of the frequency and severity of symptoms in Lyme disease patients with erythema migrans compared with matched controls at baseline, 6 months, and 12 months. Clin Infect Dis. 2020;71(12):3118–24. https://doi.org/10.1093/cid/ciz1215.
29. Steere AC. Posttreatment Lyme disease syndromes: distinct pathogenesis caused by maladaptive host responses. J Clin Invest. 2020;130(5):2148–51. https://doi.org/10.1172/JCI138062.

Pathophysiology of Early Disseminated Lyme Carditis

Shyla Gupta, Chang Nancy Wang, and Adrian Baranchuk

Abstract

Due to the presence of extra-cellular proteins, the myocardium possesses a very inviting environment for *B. burgdorferi* to adhere. This allows for a mechanism of direct invasion into the myocardial tissue, leading to cardiovascular manifestations such as myocarditis. An exaggerated inflammatory response can be seen through elevated levels of proinflammatory cytokines and deposition of the complement membrane attack complex (MAC) in patients with Lyme carditis. The maladaptive immune response to Borrelia infection is characterized by multifocal collections of T-cells, plasma cells, and macrophages. Infections often result in increased depositions of IgG and IgM in the heart. This chapter will outline the pathophysiology of early disseminated Lyme disease manifesting as Lyme carditis.

Keywords

Early disseminated Lyme carditis · Direct spirochete invasion · Proinflammatory cytokines · Inflammation · Autoimmune response

1 Introduction

Lyme disease is a bacterial infection caused by the spirochete Borrelia burgdorferi, transmitted through the bite of infected hard-bodied ticks in the genus Ixodes [1]. In the early disseminated phase of Lyme disease, the spirochete spreads into

S. Gupta (✉)
Faculty of Medicine, University of Ottawa, Ottawa, Canada
e-mail: shyladevigupta@gmail.com

C. N. Wang · A. Baranchuk
Department of Medicine, Kingston Health Sciences Center, Queen's University, Kingston, ON, Canada

various organs [2]. When Borrelia invades cardiac myocytes, this causes Lyme carditis [3]. The most common presentation of LC is high degree atrioventricular block (AVB), with less common manifestations including myocarditis, pericarditis, and arrhythmias (see Chap. 6 for details) [3]. Although Lyme carditis is a rare event affecting approximately 10% of patients with Lyme disease, the incidence of Lyme disease is increasing each year [3]. Prompt recognition of this bacterial invasion into the heart is crucial, as rapid treatment of Lyme carditis can reverse high degree AVB and prevent the need for permanent pacemaker implantation [4].

2   Method of Transmission

The stages of Lyme disease are important to differentiate to clearly understand and classify the pathophysiology of each individual phase of the disease. Firstly, spirochetes are transmitted to humans through the saliva of the ticks at the site of the bite [5]. Infection risk increases if the tick remains on the skin for at least 48 h, as this allows the bacteria to travel from the gut of the tick to its salivary glands [6]. After this initial transmission of the pathogen to the human host, Lyme disease progresses into three distinct stages: early localized, early dissemination, and late dissemination [5]. The stages of Lyme disease are described in detail in Chap. 4. In brief, the early localized phase is characterized by the appearance of erythema migrants within 3–32 days of transmission [6]. After this phase, the spirochetes spread through the circulatory and lymphatic systems to several organs throughout the body. This causes dermatological, joint, neurological, and cardiac manifestations [7]. This phase is known as the early dissemination phase and occurs days to weeks after the tick bite. The last stage, the late dissemination phase, occurs after approximately 2–3 years after pathogen transmission [5].

This chapter will focus on the specific manifestation of early disseminated Lyme carditis and the associated pathophysiology.

3   Pathophysiological Mechanisms

The pathophysiological mechanisms implicated in Lyme carditis are complex and under active study. Overarching themes of involvement include direct invasion of myocardial tissue by *B. burgdorferi*, an exaggerated inflammatory response and a maladaptive immune response (Fig. 1).

4   Direct Invasion of Myocardial Tissue by *B. Burgdorferi*

The myocardium possesses a very inviting environment for *B. burgdorferi* due to the presence of several extra-cellular proteins [8–11]. Self-adhesion to these proteins while also evading the host immune response allows for direct invasion of the myocardial tissue [12]. A study by Stanek et al. was able to isolate *B.*

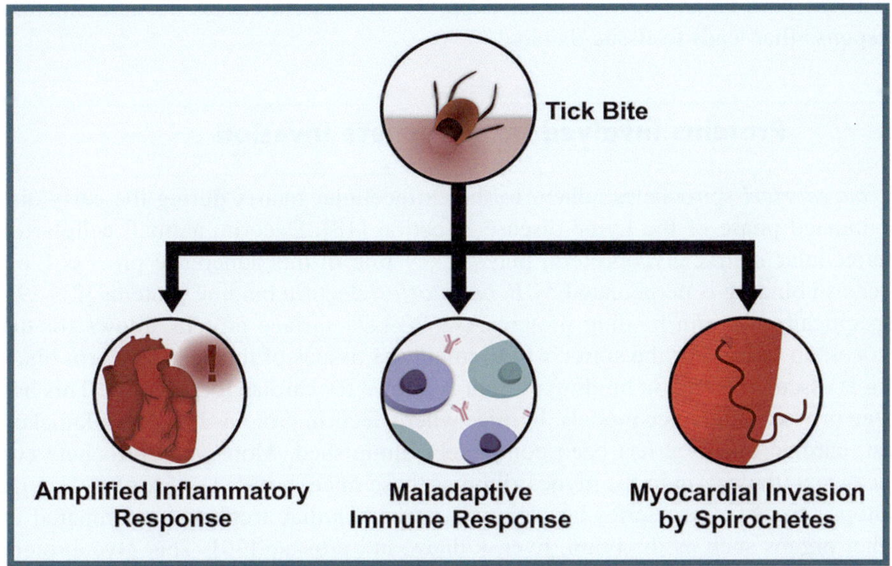

Fig. 1 Three main pathophysiological mechanisms of early disseminated Lyme Carditis include an amplified inflammatory response, maladaptive immune response and myocardial invasion by spirochetes

burgdorferi from a myocardial biopsy of a patient with Lyme carditis [13]. Histological analysis showed a characterization of enlarged, vesicular myonuclear, atrophic and hypertrophic myocardial fibers, and thickening and invasion of vessels in the endomysium by mononuclear cells.

Within the connective tissue, collagen fibers at the base of the heart, basal interventricular septum, perivascular regions, blood vessels and valves and outer and inner membranes exist [14–17]. The spirochete works to invade these structures and cause damage. Although still being investigated, research has shown that *B. burgdorferi* may also be isolated within the extracellular matrix but it does not produce any endotoxins and exotoxins [18, 19].

In early disseminated Lyme disease, myocyte necrosis is of particular concern as the endomyocardial tissue is typically impacted [20]. Moreover, between muscle fibres in the endocardium, inflammatory infiltrates are also present [20]. Amongst patients with longstanding cardiomyopathy induced by early disseminated Lyme carditis, endomyocardial biopsies have shown growth of *B. burgdorferi*. [21] Hypertrophic myocardial fibers and thickening of the walls of small endomysia vessels have also been noted [21].

Myocarditis caused by invasion of the myocardium can be a clinical manifestation alone or also in conjunction with the pericardium [22, 23]. The pathophysiology of Lyme myocarditis reveals itself to be an extensive infiltration of lymphocytes and spirochetes [8, 24]. Cross reactive antibodies react with proteins in the body, causing autoimmune injury [25]. The immunological component of Lyme carditis shows that initial exposure to bacteria causes an inflammatory response that leads to tissue damage.

5 Proteins Involved in Spirochete Invasion

B. burgdorferi spirochetes adhere to the extracellular matrix during the early disseminated phase of the Lyme disease infection [18]. Decorin, a small cellular or pericellular matrix glycoprotein, plays a key role in this adherence process [26]. Decorin binding is perpetuated by *B. burgdorferi* decorin binding proteins [27–29]. Specifically, decorin binding protein A, a 20-kDa surface protein, allows for the process to occur. For the spirochete to infect the tissues of the heart, decorin binding is essential. Decorin binding protein A allows for cardiac localization. This has been proven using mice models. In mice where decorin proteins have been knocked out, cardiac infection has been completely diminished. Moreover, spirochete co-localize with decorin in the myocardium of these mice models as observed through autopsy tissues. Case series have shown marked cardiac tropism, as compared to other organs such as the brain, liver, kidney, and prostate [30]. This glycoprotein has varied, and differential glycosaminoglycan chains attached to the protein core. Theories suggest that cardiac specific modifications of glycosaminoglycan chains alter and propagate *B. burgdorferi* spirochete adhesion in the myocardium [31, 32].

6 Exaggerated Inflammatory Response

The persistence of Borrelia or bacterial antigen in cardiac tissue causes chronic inflammation, leading to myocarditis, pericarditis, endocarditis and pancarditis [22, 33–37]. The presence of *B. burgdorferi* in the myocardium in the early disseminated phases of the disease subsequently causes processes that lead to an exaggerated inflammatory response.

Numerous studies have shown that *B. burgdorferi* can cause the release of proinflammatory cytokines, such as interleukin-1α (IL-1α), IL-1β, IL-6, IL-8, IL-12, tumor necrosis factor alpha (TNF-α), gamma interferon (IFN-γ), IL-17, granulocyte–macrophage colony-stimulating factor (GM-CSF) and IL-18 [38]. These cytokines contribute to the inflammatory response seen in Lyme carditis, which causes tissue inflammation and damage [39]. Although inflammation is important in response to tissue injury and is required for tissue repair from the invasion of spirochetes, uncontrolled inflammation results in even more tissue damage [38].

Another point of interest is BLC (also called BCA-1 or CXCL13) [39]. BLC is a chemokine that is especially selective for B-cells. BLC is characterized as a homing chemokine and has been implicated in the trafficking of lymphocytes and dendritic cells in lymphoid organs [39, 40]. Studies have found that one of the consequences of *B. burgdorferi* infection of the heart is the upregulation of BLC [16, 41–43]. This leads to infiltration of plasma cells and causes uncontrolled production and deposition of large amounts of IgM. This further exacerbates the immune response.

Another study also found deposition of the membrane attack complex (MAC) in the heart of Chagas cardiomyopathy patients [44, 45]. MACs have not only been found on spirochetes but also on the membranes of cardiac myocytes. Studies propose that MAC deposition may also add to an exaggerated immune response in early disseminated Lyme disease [16].

7 Maladaptive Immune Response

Evidenced by the above paragraphs, the pathophysiology of Lyme carditis involves direct myocardial invasion by the bacteria and inflammatory responses. Subsequent maladaptive immune processes follow, leading to further tissue damage [30].

As established, carditis is a main manifestation of early disseminated Lyme disease. More cardiac T-cells as compared to B-cells is a characterizing feature of host response during the early disseminated stage of the disease [30]. The dermal infiltrate is typically T-cells, especially found in early erythema migrants [46, 47]. B-cell infiltrates with germinal centers and evidence of pseudo clonality are also present in early disseminated Lyme disease. In European patients, it has been noted that high densities of B-cell infiltration are so alarming that the infection often mimics B-cell lymphoma [16, 48].

In mouse models during early infection states, myocardial infiltrates are made up of T-cells and very few B-cells [49]. In a nonhuman primate model of Lyme carditis, cardiac plasma cells, tissue IgG, and IgM deposition, and increased levels of the B-cell chemoattractant chemokine CXCL13 were observed in one study. In a case series, patient who were positive for Lyme IgG serology also had the greatest ratio of cardiac B0cells to T-cells [16].

Moreover, researchers have isolated dendritic cells from healthy patients and exposed them to Borrelia burgdorferi [50]. Results have shown that the bacterial infection causes receptor sites on the surface of dendritic cells, known as HLA-DRs, to mature and become active. In a typical situation, HLA-DRs cells presents antigens to killer T-cells which remove bacterial infections from the body. However, when HLA-DRs interact with Borrelia burgdorferi, they are structurally modified and prevent the dendritic cells from "marking" the bacterial proteins as foreign. This causes dendritic cells to attract T-cells, but they then attack healthy cells instead of infected cells.

Overall, there is a significant role of B- and T-cell proliferation in the early disseminated phase of Lyme carditis. The presence of cardiac T-cells is a defining characteristic of a patient with Borrelia, leading to further tissue damage. There is typically a high density of B-cell infiltration and an increased level of chemoattractant chemokines, causing a maladaptive immune response for the host.

8 Conclusions

The main pathophysiologic mechanisms of Lyme carditis can be broken down into three main points (Fig. 1). Direct spirochetal invasion of cardiac myocytes leads to myocarditis [3]. An exaggerated inflammatory response can be seen through elevated levels of proinflammatory cytokines and deposition of the complement membrane attack complex (MAC) in patients with Lyme carditis [38, 44, 45]. Finally, the maladaptive immune response to Borrelia infection is characterized by multifocal collections of T-cells, plasma cells, and macrophages [30, 49]. Infections often result in increased depositions of IgG and IgM in the heart. Overall, further elucidation needs to be conducted to determine the etiology of relapsing and persisting symptoms [51]. More research should be done to fully appreciate the presence of *B. burgdorferi* in the extracellular matrix, and the subsequent potential production of endotoxins and exotoxins [18, 19].

References

1. Wormser GP, Dattwyler RJ, Shapiro ED, et al. The clinical assessment, treatment, and prevention of Lyme disease, human granulocytic anaplasmosis, and babesiosis: clinical practice guidelines by the Infectious Diseases Society of America. Clin Infect Dis. 2006;43:1089–134.
2. Shapiro ED, Wormser GP. Lyme disease in 2018: what is new (and what is not). JAMA. 2018;320:635–6.
3. Yeung C, Baranchuk A. Diagnosis and treatment of Lyme carditis: JACC review topic of the week. J Am Coll Cardiol. 2019;73(6):717–26. https://doi.org/10.1016/j.jacc.2018.11.035.
4. Wan D, Baranchuk A. Lyme carditis and atrioventricular block. CMAJ. 2018;190:E622.
5. Tilly K, Rosa PA, Stewart PE. Biology of infection with Borrelia burgdorferi. Infect Dis Clin North Am. 2008;22(2):217–34, v. https://doi.org/10.1016/j.idc.2007.12.013.
6. Cook MJ. Lyme borreliosis: a review of data on transmission time after tick attachment. Int J Gen Med. 2014;19(8):1–8. https://doi.org/10.2147/IJGM.S73791.
7. Haddad V Jr, Haddad MR, Santos M, Cardoso JLC. Skin manifestations of tick bites in humans. An Bras Dermatol. 2018;93(2):251–5. https://doi.org/10.1590/abd1806-4841.201 86378.
8. Kubanek M, Sramko M, Berenova D, et al. Detection of Borrelia burgdorferi sensu lato in endomyocardial biopsy specimens in individuals with recent-onset dilated cardiomyopathy. Eur J Heart Fail. 2012;14:588–96.
9. Horowitz HW, Belkin RN. Acute myopericarditis resulting from Lyme disease. Am Heart J. 1995;130:176–8.
10. Maher B, Murday D, Harden SP. Cardiac MRI of Lyme disease myocarditis. Heart. 2012;98:264.
11. Palecek T, Kuchynka P, Hulinska D, et al. Presence of Borrelia burgdorferi in endomyocardial biopsies in patients with new-onset unexplained dilated cardiomyopathy. Med Microbiol Immunol. 2010;199:139–43.
12. Muehlenbachs A, Bollweg BC, Schulz TJ, et al. Cardiac tropism of Borrelia burgdorferi: an autopsy study of sudden cardiac death associated with Lyme carditis. Am J Pathol. 2016;186:1195–205.
13. Stanek G, Klein J, Bittner R, Glogar D. Isolation of Borrelia burgdorferi from the myocardium of a patient with longstanding cardiomyopathy. N Engl J Med. 1990;322:249–52.
14. Imai DM, Feng S, Hodzic E, Barthold SW. Dynamics of connective-tissue localization during chronic Borrelia burgdorferi infection. Lab Invest. 2013;93:900–10.

15. Steere AC, Batsford WP, Weinberg M, et al. Lyme carditis: cardiac abnormalities of Lyme disease. Ann Intern Med. 1980;93:8–16.
16. Cadavid D, Bai Y, Hodzic E, Narayan K, et al. Cardiac involvement in non-human primates infected with the Lyme disease spirochete Borrelia burgdorferi. Lab Invest. 2004;84:1439–50.
17. Haddad FA, Nadelman RB. Lyme disease and the heart. Front Biosci. 2003;8:s769–82.
18. Cabello FC, Godfrey HP, Newman SA. Hidden in plain sight: Borrelia burgdorferi and the extra-cellular matrix. Trends Microbiol. 2007;15:350–4.
19. Steere AC. Lyme disease. N Engl J Med. 2001;345:115–25.
20. Fish AE, Pride YB, Pinto DS. Lyme carditis. Infect Dis Clin North Am. 2008;22(2):275–88, vi. https://doi.org/10.1016/j.idc.2007.12.008.
21. Scheffold N, Herkommer B, Kandolf R, May AE. Lyme carditis–diagnosis, treatment and prognosis. Dtsch Arztebl Int. 2015;112(12):202–8. https://doi.org/10.3238/arztebl.2015.0202.
22. Yoon EC, Vail E, Kleinman G, et al. Lyme disease: a case report of a 17-year-old male with fatal Lyme carditis. Cardiovasc Pathol. 2015;24:317–21.
23. Robinson ML, Kobayashi T, Higgins Y, et al. Lyme carditis. Infect Dis Clin North Am. 2015;29:255–68.
24. Raveche ES, Schutzer SE, Fernandes H, et al. Evidence of Borrelia autoimmunity-induced component of Lyme carditis and arthritis. J Clin Microbiol. 2005;43:850–6.
25. Slifka MK, Pagarigan R, Mena I, et al. Using recombinant coxsackievirus B3 to evaluate the induction and protective efficacy of CD^{8+} T cells during picornavirus infection. J Virol. 2001;75(5):2377–87. https://doi.org/10.1128/JVI.75.5.2377-2387.2001.
26. Brown EL, Wooten RM, Johnson BJ, Iozzo RV, Smith A, Dolan MC, Guo BP, Weis JJ, Höök M. Resistance to Lyme disease in decorin-deficient mice. J Clin Invest. 2001;107(7):845–52. https://doi.org/10.1172/JCI11692.
27. Arnaboldi PM, Sambir M, Dattwyler RJ. Decorin binding proteins A and B in the serodiagnosis of Lyme disease in North America. Clin Vaccine Immunol. 2014;21(10):1426–36. https://doi.org/10.1128/CVI.00383-14.
28. Fischer JR, Parveen N, Magoun L, Leong JM. Decorin-binding proteins A and B confer distinct mammalian cell type-specific attachment by Borrelia burgdorferi, the Lyme disease spirochete. Proc Natl Acad Sci U S A. 2003;100(12):7307–12. https://doi.org/10.1073/pnas.1231043100.
29. Lin YP, Benoit V, Yang X, et al. Strain-specific variation of the decorin-binding adhesin DbpA influences the tissue tropism of the Lyme disease spirochete. PLoS Pathog. 2014;10(7):e1004238. https://doi.org/10.1371/journal.ppat.1004238.
30. Muehlenbachs A, Bollweg BC, Schulz TJ, et al. Cardiac tropism of Borrelia burgdorferi: an autopsy study of sudden cardiac death associated with Lyme Carditis. Am J Pathol. 2016;186(5):1195–205. https://doi.org/10.1016/j.ajpath.2015.12.027.
31. Antonara S, Ristow L, Coburn J. Adhesion mechanisms of Borrelia burgdorferi. Adv Exp Med Biol. 2011;715:35–49. https://doi.org/10.1007/978-94-007-0940-9_3.
32. Kumar D, Ristow LC, Shi M, et al. Intravital imaging of vascular transmigration by the Lyme spirochete: requirement for the integrin binding residues of the B. burgdorferi P66 protein. PLoS Pathog. 2015;11(12):e1005333. https://doi.org/10.1371/journal.ppat.1005333.
33. van der Linde MR. Lyme carditis: clinical characteristics of 105 cases. Scand J Infect Dis Suppl. 1991;77:81–4.
34. Pinto DS. Cardiac manifestations of Lyme dis- ease. Med Clin North Am. 2002;86:285–96.
35. Manzoor K, Aftab W, Choksi S, Khan IA. Lyme carditis: sequential electrocardiographic changes in response to antibiotic therapy. Int J Cardiol. 2009;137:167–71.
36. Bush LM, Vazquez-Pertejo MT. Tick borne illness-Lyme disease. Dis Mon. 2018;64:195–212.
37. Ciesielski CA, Markowitz LE, Horsley R, et al. Lyme disease surveillance in the United States, 1983–1986. Rev Infect Dis 1989;11 Suppl 6:S1435–41.
38. Dennis VA, Jefferson A, Singh SR, et al. Interleukin-10 anti-inflammatory response to Borrelia burgdorferi, the agent of Lyme disease: a possible role for suppressors of cytokine signaling 1 and 3. Infect Immun. 2006;74(10):5780–9. https://doi.org/10.1128/IAI.00678-06.

39. Giambartolomei GH, Dennis VA, Lasater BL, Philipp MT. Induction of pro- and anti-inflammatory cytokines by Borrelia burgdorferi lipoproteins in monocytes is mediated by CD14. Infect Immun. 1999;67(1):140–7. https://doi.org/10.1128/IAI.67.1.140-147.1999.
40. Hjelmström P, Fjell J, Nakagawa T, et al. Lymphoid tissue homing chemokines are expressed in chronic inflammation. Am J Pathol. 2000;156(4):1133–8. https://doi.org/10.1016/S0002-9440(10)64981-4.
41. Ruddle NH. Lymphoid neo-organogenesis: lymphotoxin's role in inflammation and development. Immunol Res. 1999;19:119–25.
42. Amft N, Curnow SJ, Scheel-Toellner D, et al. Ectopic expression of the B cell-attracting chemokine BCA-1 (CXCL13) on endothelial cells and within lymphoid follicles contributes to the establishment of germinal center-like structures in Sjogren's syndrome. Arthritis Rheum. 2001;44:2633–41.
43. Pachner AR, Dail D, Narayan K, et al. Increased expression of B-lymphocyte chemoattractant, but not pro-inflammatory cytokines, in muscle tissue in rhesus chronic Lyme borreliosis. Cytokine. 2002;19:297–307.
44. Aiello VD, Reis MM, Benvenuti LA, et al. A possible role for complement in the pathogenesis of chronic chagasic cardiomyopathy. J Pathol. 2002;197:224–9.
45. Yasojima K, Schwab C, McGeer EG, et al. Human heart generates complement proteins that are upregulated and activated after myocardial infarction. Circ Res. 1998;83:860–9.
46. Büchner SA, Rufli T. Erythema chronicum migrans: evidence for cellular immune reaction in the skin lesion. Dermatologica. 1987;174(3):144–9. https://doi.org/10.1159/000249007.
47. Ma Y, Bramwell KK, Lochhead RB, et al. Borrelia burgdorferi arthritis-associated locus Bbaa1 regulates Lyme arthritis and K/B×N serum transfer arthritis through intrinsic control of type I IFN production. J Immunol. 2014;193(12):6050–60. https://doi.org/10.4049/jimmunol.1401746.
48. Grange F, Wechsler J, Guillaume JC, et al. Borrelia burgdorferi-associated lymphocytoma cutis simulating a primary cutaneous large B-cell lymphoma. J Am Acad Dermatol. 2002;47(4):530–4. https://doi.org/10.1067/mjd.2002.120475.
49. Ruderman EM, Kerr JS, Telford SR III, et al. Early murine Lyme carditis has a macrophage predominance and is independent of major histocompatibility complex class II-CD^{4+} T cell interactions. J Infect Dis. 1995;171(2):362–70. https://doi.org/10.1093/infdis/171.2.362.
50. Gutierrez-Hoffmann MG, O'Meally RN, Cole RN, et al. Borrelia burgdorferi-induced changes in the class II self-Immunopeptidome displayed on HLA-DR molecules expressed by dendritic cells. Front Med (Lausanne). 2020;16(7):568. https://doi.org/10.3389/fmed.2020.00568.
51. Donta ST. What we know and don't know about Lyme disease. Front Public Health. 2022;21(9):819541. https://doi.org/10.3389/fpubh.2021.819541.

Clinical Manifestations of Early Disseminated Lyme Carditis

Andres F. Miranda-Arboleda, Juan G. Sierra-David, Rachel Wamboldt, and Adrian Baranchuk

Abstract

Atrioventricular conduction abnormalities are the most common presentation of early disseminated Lyme carditis. Up to two-thirds of patients with Lyme carditis will progress to a high-degree atrioventricular block; however, it can reverse completely when early antibiotic treatment is provided. A systematic approach to early disseminated Lyme carditis is essential since the identification of Lyme as the etiology in patients with heart block will avoid the unnecessary implantation of permanent pacemakers. This chapter covers the clinical manifestation of early disseminated Lyme carditis.

Keywords

Early disseminated Lyme carditis • Atrioventricular blocks • SILC Score • Myocarditis • Pancarditis

1 Introduction

Lyme Disease (LD) is a zoonosis caused most typically by the gram-negative spirochete *Borrelia burgdorferi* sensu lato complex, transmitted by the Ixodes-thick. There are other less common types of Borrelia such as *B. garinii, B. afzelii,* and *B. spielmanii* which can also cause the disease. LD is the most commonly reported vector-borne disease in North America accounting for approximately 80% of tick-borne diseases reported in the US [1, 2]. In Canada, the number of LD cases has

A. F. Miranda-Arboleda (✉) · R. Wamboldt · A. Baranchuk
Division of Cardiology, Queen's University-Kingston Health Sciences Centre, Kingston, ON, Canada
e-mail: andreas.miranda@queensu.ca

J. G. Sierra-David
Division of Cardiology, Naples Heart Institute-Naples Healthcare System, Naples, FL, USA

A. Baranchuk et al. (eds.), *Lyme Carditis*,
https://doi.org/10.1007/978-3-031-41169-4_6

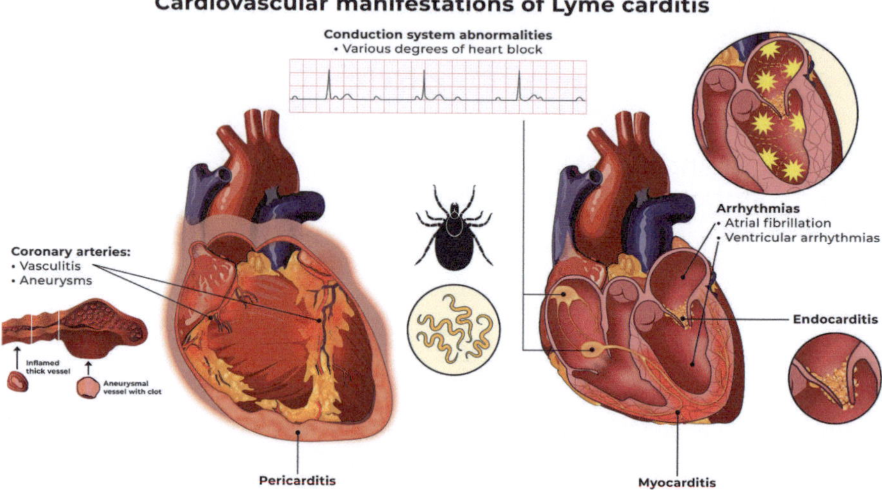

Fig. 1 Cardiovascular manifestations of early disseminated Lyme disease

climbed steadily, and risk modeling suggests that cases will continue to increase due to *I. scapularis,* as this tick is carried by migratory birds that are affected by climate change and will invade further into southern Canada [3, 4].

Early Disseminated Lyme Disease (EDLD) represents the stage when bacteria spreads to other organs and it may have cutaneous, cardiovascular, musculoskeletal, neurological, and/or ocular complications. Cardiac manifestations also called Lyme carditis (LC), are present in approximately 10% of patients with LD. The onset of LC typically occurs within one to two months after exposure as a form of EDLD. The most common type of cardiac involvement is atrioventricular block (AVB) which occurs in about 90% of patients hospitalized with LC [1]. Children mostly manifest carditis and myocardial involvement, and up to 30% have electrocardiographic (ECG) changes [5] (Fig. 1).

The purpose of this chapter is to describe the cardiovascular manifestations of patients with early disseminated Lyme carditis and provide a stepwise diagnostic algorithm.

2   Pathophysiology

Following the inoculation of *Borrelia sp.* in the skin by the tick, the spirochete invades subcutaneous tissue, and due to its marked tropism for the heart tissue advances via the bloodstream to the myocardium infiltrating collagen fibers in the extracellular matrix provoking an inflammatory response by the host [6]. Approximately two to three weeks after initial infection, evidence of this bacteria can be found in higher concentrations in the AV junction, however, other cardiac structures such as the atrial root, atrial and ventricular myocardium, endocardium, myocardium, and the perivascular spaces can also be affected [6, 7].

The immunologic response is predominantly cellular and mediated by macrophages and lymphocytes which cause collateral damage to the cardiac structures and is responsible for most of the cardiac manifestations of LC. The valves or blood vessels are rarely affected in LC, and therefore, although previously described, it is uncommon to see valvular abnormalities or vasculitis as a clinical manifestation [7].

It is not currently known whether the borrelia spirochete can produce endo or exotoxins. However, cytokine release is facilitated by the phagocytosis of the bacteria, triggering the activation of natural killer cells, and generating a vicious circle of inflammation and tissue injury [7]. Increased immunogenicity can contribute to the LC pathophysiology. This is suggested by the presence of a few spirochetes causing significant lymphocytic myocardial infiltration in the absence of toxin or cell invasion [7].

Autoimmunity has been suggested to play a role in EDLC [8]. Research by *Raveche* et al., found that Borrelia protein OspA has properties of molecular mimicry in mice, and it can generate cross-reactivity against myosin. Self-component cross-reactivity can be important in future exposition that may react with self-constituents [8].

3 Clinical Findings—Early Disseminated Lyme Carditis (EDLC)

3.1 General Symptoms

Many patients with LC do not recall a tick bite. LD is primarily a clinical diagnosis, and a high index of suspicion is required. There is a small predominance of males. General symptoms and limited disease after the *Ixodes* tick have bitten the host are more common. Patients often present with erythema migrans, and general constitutional symptoms such as fever, fatigue, chills, and arthralgia (Table 1).

3.2 Atrioventricular Conduction Abnormalities

The most common manifestation is the atrioventricular block (AVB) in 90% of admitted patients with LC, and approximately 60% of those progress to high-degree AVB which is transient, and most often supra-hisian, in which conduction delays originate above the Bundle of His. The duration of AVB can last minutes, hours, or days. Other less common conduction or rhythm alterations include the presence of sinus node disease, atrial fibrillation, supraventricular tachycardia, ventricular tachycardia, fibrillation, and intraventricular conduction abnormalities [6] (Fig. 1).

Table 1 Clinical Manifestations of Lyme carditis

General signs and symptoms	Frequency reported, %
Documented rash	54
Fever	43
Fatigue/Malaise	39.8
Cardiovascular signs and symptoms	
Presyncope	63
Syncope	33
Shortness of breath	3
Extracardiac manifestations	
Arthralgia	23
Cranial neuritis	10
Arthritis	3
Meningitis	3
Electrocardiographic findings	
Third-degree Atrioventricular block	77.3
Second-degree Atrioventricular block	33.0
Asystole/Sinus Pauses	12.5
Resolution	
Atrioventricular block resolved	94.3

Modified from Besant G, Wan D, Yeung C, et al. Suspicious index in Lyme carditis: Systematic review and proposed new risk score. Clin Cardiol Dec 2018;41:1611–1616 and Shen RV, McCarthy CA, Smith RP. Lyme Carditis in Hospitalized Children and Adults, a Case Series. Open Forum Infect Dis Jul 2021;8:ofab140 [5, 15]

Progression from mild forms of AV block (first-degree or second-degree Mobitz I) to more advanced presentations (second-degree Mobitz II, high degree or complete heart block) in patients with LC may occur rapidly and patients need to be monitored closely in the hospital until evidence of conduction recovers is observed[9, 10].

Many factors are relevant when considering high-degree AVB in patients with LC;

(1) It is a common presentation of this disease.
(2) It is transient, particularly when timely treated with antibiotics.
(3) The standard treatment of high-degree AVB due to other etiologies, once correctable causes have been ruled out, is the insertion of a permanent pacing device.
(4) LC mostly affects young patients who will embark in a whole life engagement process with a permanent pacemaker that might be not needed [1, 6, 11, 12].

In that sense, identifying whether a high-degree AV block is caused by LC is of critical importance, and requires the appropriate clinical context, and a high suspicion index.

3.3 Myocarditis/Pericarditis

EDLC can also present with acute myocarditis, pericarditis, myopericarditis, endocarditis as well as pancarditis, and can mimic acute coronary syndromes. ST segment depression and T wave inversion in the inferolateral leads can be seen in up to 60% and remit after antibiotic therapy (Fig. 1). It has been hypothesized that some of the improvements in left ventricular dysfunction attributed to transient conduction system disease, have been identified in patients with LD [1, 6].

3.4 Miscellaneous Abnormalities

Case reports have described other uncommon manifestations of LC such as valve endocarditis, cardiogenic shock, and arteritis. (Fig. 1) [6, 13, 14]. However, their diagnosis is difficult due to the high suspicion index required to diagnose them and their high mortality rate.

4 Diagnosis

Our group, in publications led by *Besant* and *Yeung* et al. [15, 16] proposed the use of the Suspicious Index in Lime Carditis (SILC) score as a systematic approach to patients presenting with HDAVB, aiming to early identify those at risk of LC to provide quick antibiotic treatment and postpone the implantation of permanent pacemakers (Fig. 2).

The SILC score components are summarized by the mnemonic COSTAR:

- Constitutional symptoms; fever, malaise: 2 points
- Outdoor activity: 1 point
- Sex; Male: 1 point
- Tick bite: 3 points
- Age < 50 years: 1 point
- Rash; Erythema migrans: 4 points.

A score 0–2 represents a low risk of HDAVB being caused by LC, 3–6 intermediate and, 7–12 a high risk, respectively (Table 2) [15]. If a SILC Score is low (0–2), no further testing is needed and if considered appropriate patients presenting with HDAVB can proceed with permanent pacemaker implantation. Whereas if the SILC score is 3 or more, *B. burgdorferi* serology testing with ELISA and/or Western Blot is warranted, and antibiotic therapy should be started immediately until the test results are available[15, 16]. For a more detailed review of the SILC score please refer to Chap. 7 of this book.

Serological testing includes ELISA to identify IgM or IgG antibodies against *B. burgdorferi*. Certain caveats need to be accounted for: false negative testing secondary to delayed immune response, this does not necessarily rule out LC.

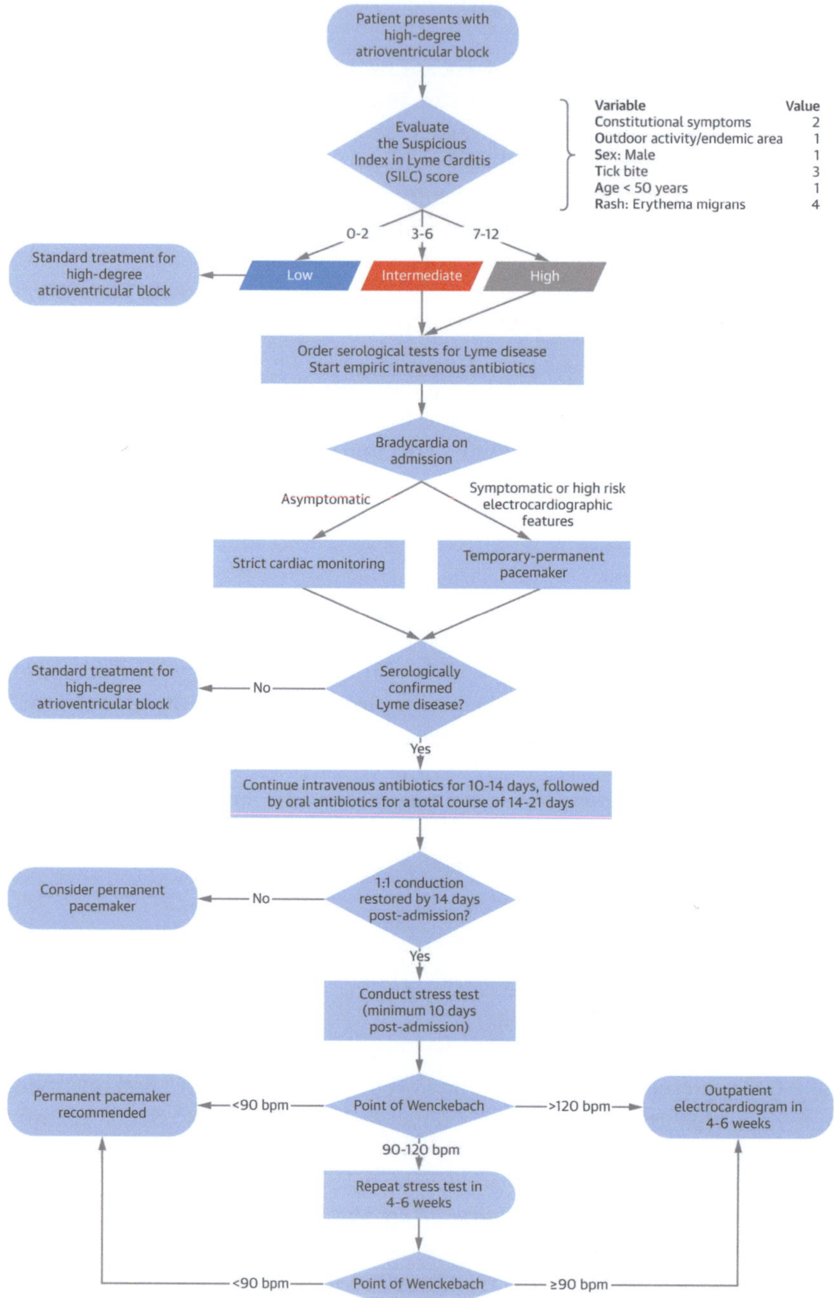

Fig. 2 A systematic approach to High-degree AV block in the setting of Lyme carditis. Reproduced with permission from this manuscript: Yeung C, Baranchuk A. Systematic Approach to the Diagnosis and Treatment of Lyme Carditis and High-Degree Atrioventricular Block. Healthcare (Basel) Sep 22 2018;6(16). Copyright Elsevier (2023)

Table 2 Suspicious index in Lyme carditis (SILC) score[a]

Variable	Value
Constitutional symptoms (malaise, fever)	2
Outdoor activity/endemic area	1
Sex = Male	1
Tick bite	3
Age < 50 years old	1
Rash = Erythema migrans	4

Interpretation: Low risk score: 0–2, Intermediate risk score: 3–6, High-risk score: 7–12

[a] Besant G, Wan D, Yeung C, et al. Suspicious index in Lyme carditis: Systematic review and proposed new risk score. Clin Cardiol Dec 2018;41:1611–1616[15]

On the other hand, positive serologies especially IgG may reflect a prior remote infection and therefore may not be the cause of the HDAVB in patients presenting without other symptoms of LC. A two-tiered approach usually involves an initial ELISA as a screening and if the results are positive or indeterminate a Western Blot can confirm the diagnosis. Of note, sensitivity significantly increases when extracutaneous manifestations such as LC are present (87–100%) [9].

Additional cardiac testing may be needed depending on the LC presentation. Abnormal echocardiographic findings may include left or right ventricular dilatations and involvement of the left and ventricular function as a sign of myocarditis. Cardiac magnetic resonance imaging (MRI) may show signs of inflammation such as myocardial wall edema, either acute such as decreased signal intensity or subacute to chronic represented by late gadolinium enhancement with subendocardial sparing. Pericardial inflammation can be seen either on an echocardiogram or in MRI [1, 6, 17]. Our group uses exercise stress testing before discharge to prove recovery of 1:1 atrioventricular conduction at faster heart rates before discharge in selected patients admitted initially with HDAVB.

5 Treatment

Prevention is the cornerstone of the treatment of LC, most of the LD cases occur between June and December (in North America), therefore preventive strategies to minimize tick exposure should be adopted while doing outdoor activities. Wearing protective clothing such as long-sleeve shirts, and long pants; use repellent and adoption of a tick check and removal habitude after potential exposure to ticks. In the case of tick detection, it has been proved that during the first 72 h of a tick attachment, one dose of doxycycline decreases the chance of LD by approximately 90% [1, 3, 9].

Antibiotics are the cornerstone of LC treatment because their early initiation reduces the length of the symptoms and the risk of additional complications [18].

Based on the systematic approach to LC mentioned above [15, 16], in patients with SILC intermediate or high it is recommended to start intravenous antibiotics once the suspicion of LC rises and while the serology and additional cardiovascular test are obtained [15]. Ceftriaxone is the most used parenteral antibiotic for LC, it is usually administered during the hospital for 7–10 days until conduction abnormalities improved (1:1 AV conduction, PR interval < 300 ms) [1, 18]. Other parenteral antibiotic alternatives include Cefotaxime and Penicillin G (Table 3) [18]. Once conduction abnormalities have subsided, temporary pacemakers are removed, and LC patients can be transitioned to oral antibiotics to complete 14–21 days of total treatment time. Doxycycline is the standard oral antibiotic in adults, alternative options include amoxicillin, phenoxymethylpenicillin, cefuroxime, and azithromycin (Table 3) [1, 18]. Extended courses of antibiotics have not been translated into better outcomes and they may imply higher costs and risks of adverse effects [9].

The use of temporary pacing is the gold standard for patients who develop symptomatic high-degree AVB, depending on every center's expertise this can be achieved through temporary floating wires or temporary-permanent pacemakers. The biggest advantage of temporary-permanent pacemakers is their higher stability in position and threshold over the days and the fact that they allow earlier patient mobilization as has been previously reported in our center experience [12].

A deliberate implant of permanent pacemakers is not recommended in patients with LC because most of the patients recover conduction even weeks after their

Table 3 Commonly used antibiotics in patients with Lyme carditis

Drug	Adult dose	Pediatric dose
Parenteral medications[a]		
Ceftriaxone	2 g IV once daily	50–70 mg/kg IV once daily[b]
Cefotaxime	2 g IV every 8 h	150–200 mg/kg per day divided into three–four daily doses[c]
Penicillin G	18–24 million units IV per day divided into six daily doses	250 000–400 000 U/kg per day divided into six daily doses IV[d]
Oral medications[e]		
Doxycycline	100 mg two times a day	≥ 8 years—4 mg/kg per day divided into two doses a day
Amoxicillin	500 mg three times a day	50 mg/kg per day divided into three doses a day
Cefuroxime axetil	500 mg two times a day	30 mg/kg per day divided into two daily doses
Azithromycin	500 mg once daily	10 mg/kg per day

IV: intravenously

[a] usually given during the first seven to ten days, [b] Maximum dose: 2 g IV daily, [c] Maximum dose: 6 g daily, [d] Maximum dose = 18–24 million units per day, [e] transition when the parenteral scheme is finished, usually given until competition of 14–21 days of the antibiotic course

initial presentation [1]. In a recent single-center observational study from Canada, Wang et al. showed that after 20 months of follow-up, all patients resolved AV conduction abnormalities, and none of them were on permanent pacing at discharge [12]. Permanent pacing is not usually recommended in LC unless conduction abnormalities persist despite adequate antibiotic therapy for at least three weeks [5].

6 Prognosis

LC can resolve spontaneously; however, since LC result from the dissemination of the bacteria to the cardiac structures and tissues, the early use of antibiotic therapy may help to shorten this period and its related complications [11, 19].

Once antibiotic therapy is initiated, the time to reach a PR interval of less than 300 ms, as a marker of progressive resolution of AV conduction disturbances has been established in an average of four days [5]. Occasionally LC may last up to six weeks before it recovers completely [9].

The self-limited nature of conduction abnormalities in LC has permitted consideration of the possibility of early pacemaker extraction in patients for whom the main indication of pacing was AVB in the context of LC. A recent case series described the successful explantation of permanent pacemakers in patients with previous LC. This raises the importance of detailed clinical analysis before definite pacing is considered in Lyme patients and highlighting the role of early device interrogation after implant to define possible device extraction, in order to avoid the long-term effects and complications associated with pacemakers [20].

The association of LC and chronic dilated cardiomyopathy is still a matter of controversy. Possible untreated or partially treated cases of LC may evolve into permanent myocardial dysfunction. A meta-analysis published by Motamed et al. concluded that current evidence suggests a role of chronic *Borrelia sp.* infection as a potential etiology of dilated cardiomyopathy, however, additional research needs to be performed in this field. A deeper analysis of the long-term cardiovascular complications of LC is provided in Chap. 14 of this book [19].

Previous series have reported cases of fatal presentation in LD, those cases have been mainly associated with fulminant myocarditis or coronary arteries affection; however mortality is an uncommon complication in this disease (5, 21).

7 Conclusion

Lyme carditis is a potential complication of early disseminated Lyme disease. It can affect almost any structure of the heart, but atrioventricular conduction abnormalities are the most common presentation. Atrioventricular block in Lyme carditis is a potentially reversible condition, therefore a systematic approach to identifying *B. burgdorferi* as the etiology of high-degree AVB will facilitate the early initiation of antibiotic therapy, temporary pacemakers, and ultimately minimize the unnecessary implantation of permanent pacemakers with their potential long-term implications.

References

1. Yeung C, Baranchuk A. Diagnosis and treatment of Lyme Carditis: JACC review topic of the week. J Am Coll Cardiol. 2019;73(6):717–26.
2. Centers for Disease Control and Prevention. Lyme disease: data and surveillance. 2022 [cited 2022 Nov 11]. Available from: www.cdc.gov/lyme/stats/index.html.
3. Public Health Agency of Canada. Surveillance of Lyme disease. 2022 [cited 2022 Nov 11]. Available from: https://www.canada.ca/en/public-health/services/diseases/lyme-disease/survei llance-lyme-disease.html.
4. Ripoche M, Gasmi S, Adam-Poupart A, Koffi JK, Lindsay LR, Ludwig A, et al. Passive tick surveillance provides an accurate early signal of emerging Lyme disease risk and human cases in Southern Canada. J Med Entomol. 2018;55(4):1016–26.
5. Shen RV, McCarthy CA, Smith RP. Lyme Carditis in hospitalized children and adults, a case series. Open Forum Infect Dis. 2021;8(7):ofab140.
6. Robinson ML, Kobayashi T, Higgins Y, Calkins H, Melia MT. Lyme carditis. Infect Dis Clin North Am. 2015;29(2):255–68.
7. Montgomery RR, Booth CJ, Wang X, Blaho VA, Malawista SE, Brown CR. Recruitment of macrophages and polymorphonuclear leukocytes in Lyme carditis. Infect Immun. 2007;75(2):613–20.
8. Raveche ES, Schutzer SE, Fernandes H, Bateman H, McCarthy BA, Nickell SP, et al. Evidence of Borrelia autoimmunity-induced component of Lyme carditis and arthritis. J Clin Microbiol. 2005;43(2):850–6.
9. Krause PJ, Bockenstedt LK. Cardiology patient pages. Lyme disease and the heart. Circulation. 2013;127(7):e451–4.
10. Uzomah UA, Rozen G, Mohammadreza Hosseini S, Shaqdan A, Ledesma PA, Yu X, et al. Incidence of carditis and predictors of pacemaker implantation in patients hospitalized with Lyme disease. PLoS ONE. 2021;16(11):e0259123.
11. van der Linde MR. Lyme carditis: clinical characteristics of 105 cases. Scand J Infect Dis Suppl. 1991;77:81–4.
12. Wang CN, Yeung C, Enriquez A, Chacko S, Hanson S, Redfearn D, et al. Long-term outcomes in treated Lyme Carditis. Curr Probl Cardiol. 2022;47(10):100939.
13. Fatima B, Sohail MR, Schaff HV. Lyme disease-an unusual cause of a mitral valve endocarditis. Mayo Clin Proc Innov Qual Outcomes. 2018;2(4):398–401.
14. Duray PH. Histopathology of clinical phases of human Lyme disease. Rheum Dis Clin North Am. 1989;15(4):691–710.
15. Besant G, Wan D, Yeung C, Blakely C, Branscombe P, Suarez-Fuster L, et al. Suspicious index in Lyme carditis: systematic review and proposed new risk score. Clin Cardiol. 2018;41(12):1611–6.
16. Yeung C, Baranchuk A. Systematic approach to the diagnosis and treatment of Lyme Carditis and high-degree atrioventricular block. Healthcare (Basel). 2018;6(4).
17. Munk PS, Orn S, Larsen AI. Lyme carditis: persistent local delayed enhancement by cardiac magnetic resonance imaging. Int J Cardiol. 2007;115(3):e108–10.
18. Stanek G, Wormser GP, Gray J, Strle F. Lyme borreliosis. Lancet. 2012;379(9814):461–73.
19. Motamed M, Liblik K, Miranda-Arboleda AF, Wamboldt R, Wang CN, Cingolani O, et al. Disseminated Lyme disease and dilated cardiomyopathy: a systematic review. Trends Cardiovasc Med. 2022.
20. Wamboldt R, Wang CN, Miller JC, Enriquez A, Yeung C, Chacko S, et al. Pacemaker explanation in patients with Lyme Carditis. JACC Case Rep. 2022;4(10):613–6.

21. Muehlenbachs A, Bollweg BC, Schulz TJ, Forrester JD, DeLeon CM, Molins C, et al. Cardiac tropism of Borrelia burgdorferi: an autopsy study of sudden cardiac death associated with Lyme Carditis. Am J Pathol. 2016;186(5):1195–205.

Differential Diagnosis of Unexpected Atrioventricular Blocks and Application of the SILC Score

Göksel Çinier, Rachel Wamboldt, and Juan Farina

Abstract

Atrioventricular blocks (AVBs) are described as the sudden loss of otherwise normal 1:1 atrioventricular (AV) conduction, commonly caused by ischemic heart disease, drugs, electrolyte disturbances and iatrogenic procedures and systemic illness. Advanced conduction abnormalities are treated with a permanent pacemaker in the absence of a clear reversible cause. In regions endemic for Lyme disease, Lyme carditis as a cause of reversible AVB must be ruled out to avoid the unnecessary insertion of a permanent pacemaker.

Keywords

Lyme carditis · Heart block · Lyme disease · Pacemaker

1 Introduction

Atrioventricular blocks (AVBs) are described as the sudden loss of otherwise normal 1:1 atrioventricular (AV) conduction. AVBs are most commonly encountered in older individuals as a result of the degeneration of the cardiac conduction tissue and are associated with significant morbidity and mortality. In the absence of a reversible cause, advanced conduction abnormalities are effectively treated with a permanent pacemaker. AVBs are infrequently observed in younger, otherwise

G. Çinier (✉) · J. Farina
Department of Cardiac Electrophysiology, Basaksehir Cam and Sakura City Hospital, Istanbul, Turkey
e-mail: ciniergoksel@gmail.com

R. Wamboldt · J. Farina
Department of Cardiology, Kingston Health Sciences Centre, Queen's University, Kingston, Canada
e-mail: 17reaw@queensu.ca

© The Author(s), under exclusive license to Springer Nature Switzerland AG 2023 69
A. Baranchuk et al. (eds.), *Lyme Carditis*,
https://doi.org/10.1007/978-3-031-41169-4_7

healthy individuals. One prospective cohort study using the UK Biobank found an increasing frequency of conduction disorders with age [1]. In males, they found the prevalence of conduction system diseases to be 0.16% for those aged < 55 years, 0.42% for those aged 55–64 years and 0.78% for those above the age of 65 years [1]. In females, the rates of conduction system disease was 0.08% in those aged < 55 years, 0.19% for those aged 55–64 years and 0.34% for those over the age of 65 years [1]. The loss of 1:1 AV conduction can be due to a primary abnormality of the cardiac conduction system or a secondary manifestation of another systemic disease. Patients may be completely asymptomatic or suffer severe cardiac symptoms such as fatigue, palpitations, presyncope or syncope, in addition to those symptoms associated with concomitant systemic disease.

AVB should be rapidly recognized so that timely investigations and intervention can occur. The most common causes of AVB include ischemic heart disease, drugs, electrolyte disturbances and iatrogenic, amongst others (table 1). Careful consideration of the etiology of AVB is important as some of the causes are potentially reversible, and do not require the placement of a permanent pacemaker. If necessary, patients with reversible high-grade AVB can be treated with transvenous temporary pacemakers or temporary-permanent pacing devices. The unnecessary implantation of a permanent pacemaker, besides being a significant healthcare expense, only cures the consequence of the disease, not the underlying cause.

In regions that are endemic to Lyme disease (LD), infection with *Borrelia burgdorferi* must be ruled out before considering implantation of a permanent pacemaker. Timely initiation of antibiotics can prevent progression to high grade AVB in patients presenting with cardiac conduction abnormalities, even while awaiting the results of serological testing. In addition to Lyme carditis (LC) there are many other causes of unexpected AVB, which we will briefly describe in this chapter.

2   Brief Anatomy and Physiology of the Atrioventricular Junction

The atrioventricular node (AVN) is a structure located just beneath the right atrial endocardium, at the apex of the Koch triangle. This anatomical triangle is bordered anteriorly by the insertion of the septal leaflet of the tricuspid valve, posteriorly by the Tendon of Todoro and basally by the ostium of the coronary sinus (CS). AV conduction continues through penetrating Bundle of His perforating the central fibrous body (CFB) which consists of right fibrous trigone and membranous part of the interventricular septum [2]. The penetrating bundle of His then divides into the left and right branches.

The area of the AVN is highly innervated by adrenergic and cholinergic fibers. Dromotropy is defined as the rate of electrical conduction in the cardiac tissue. Adrenergic fibers cause activation of L type Ca^{++} channels leading to a positive dromotropic effect, while cholinergic fibers cause a negative dromotropic effect, through activation of inward rectifying K^+ channels. The impact of the sympathetic

Table 1 Differential diagnosis for atrioventricular heart block

Congenital	Acquired Tranient	Acquired Persistent
• **Physiologic-** Carotid hypersensitivity, athletic training, sleep, pain • **Vasovagal** • Congenital heart disease • Maternal SLE • Progressive familiar heart block (Type IA, IB, II) • **Neuromuscular disorders**—Myotonic dystrophy, Becker muscular dystrophy, Kearns-Sayre syndrome, Erb dystrophy, Peroneal muscular dystrophy	• **Infection-** Lyme disease • **Acute ischemia or infarction** • **Metabolic-** Hyperkalemia, hypothyroidism, hypomagnesemia, adrenal insufficiency • **Drugs-** Calcium channel blockers, beta blockers, digoxin, procainamide, quinidine, anti-psychotics, TCAs, lithium • **Toxins-** Cocaine, organophosphates	• **Degenerative-** Lev's disease • **Acute ischemia or infarction** • **Toxins-** Alcohol • **Infiltrative-** Sarcoidosis, amyloidosis, hemochromatosis • **Inflammatory-** Rheumatic fever, Kawasaki's disease, reactive arthritis, ankylosing spondylitis, lupus, systemic sclerosis • **Infection-** Endocarditis, myocarditis, syphilis, Chagas' disease, tuberculosis, diphtheria, toxoplasmosis, AIDS, COVID-19 • **Neoplastic-** Lymphoma, mesothelioma, melanoma • **Iatrogenic-** Radiation, catheter ablation

and parasympathetic system is predominant in the AVN area rather than the His bundle region.

AV block is defined as delayed or complete interruption of AV nodal conduction and is classically divided into first, second and third- degree (complete) block. First-degree AV block is defined as a prolonged PR interval of more than 0.20 s. Second-degree, type I AV block involves progressive PR prolongation until one QRS "drops out", while second- degree, type II AV block is characterized by a constant PR interval before and after a blocked QRS beat. Third-degree AV block or complete heart block is defined as a complete interruption of AV conduction [3].

3 Causes of Atrioventricular Block

The causes of AVB can be classified into three major groups; (1) Congenital or inherited AVB, (2) Acquired transient AVB and (3) Acquired persistent AVB (Table 1). The major focus of this chapter is "unexpected causes of AVB"; therefore, congenital and common acquired causes of AVB will not be discussed. Instead, we will detail specific unexpected causes of AVB that should be considered when young, otherwise healthy individual present with new AVB (Table 1).

4 Infectious Diseases

Several infectious agents are known to cause AVB in the acute or chronic phases of the diseases including LD, rheumatic fever, Chagas disease, acquired immunodeficiency syndrome (AIDS), tuberculosis and recently coronavirus disease 19 (COVID-19). Involvement of the myocardial tissue is the underlying mechanism for the cardiac rhythm disturbances in majority of the cases.

4.1 *Lyme Disease*

The most common presentation of LC is AVB in 90% of cases, with high-grade AVB is observed in approximately two-thirds of cases [4, 5]. The degree of AVB seen in LC can fluctuate and progress rapidly from simple prolongation of the PR interval to His-Purkinje blocks (Fig. 1). High-grade AVB is the most common presentation of LC and often responds to antibiotic therapy. High-grade AVB typically resolves with antibiotic therapy within 10 days and mild conduction disturbances within 6 weeks [6]. Patients with first-degree AV block following Lyme disease have a much higher risk of progression when the PQ interval is above 300 ms [7]. Further details surrounding the clinical presentation of LC can be found in further detail in Chap. 6.

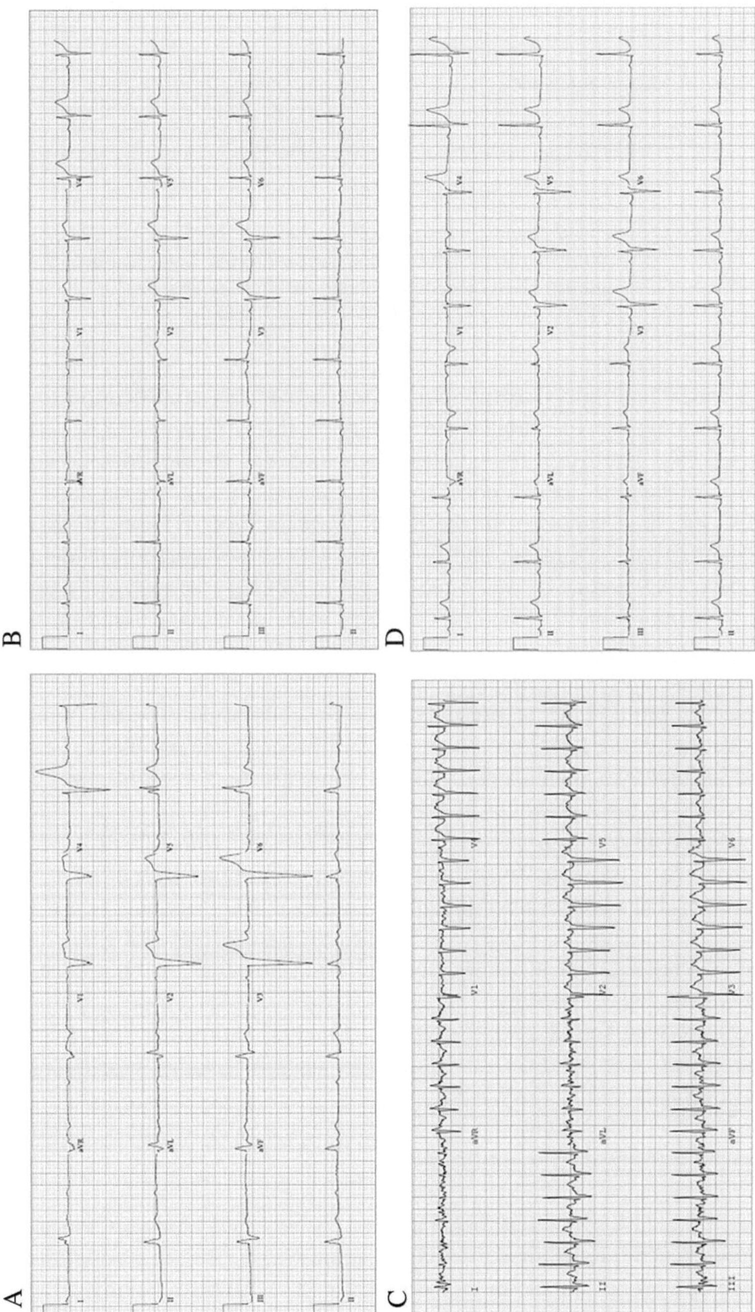

Fig. 1 Natural evolution of atrioventricular conduction abnormalities in a patient with Lyme carditis on antibiotic treatment. A 32-year-old man, military worker, presented with non-prodromal syncope. He had no cardiovascular history, but had erythema migrans, constitutional symptoms and high-risk outdoor activities on questioning, giving him a SILC score of 9 points. He reported no recollection of a tick bite. Serial 12-lead ECGs depict; **a** Complete heart block on arrival with an infra-Hisian escape; **b** 1:1 atrioventricular conduction before discharge after 10 days of intravenous antibiotics; **c** Exercise stress test with 1:1 atrioventricular conduction at a heart rate of 160 BPM before discharge; **d** Normal ECG 30 days after discharge. BPM: beats per minute, CV: cardiovascular, ECG: electrocardiogram, SILC: Suspicious Index in Lyme Carditis

Table 2 The suspicious index in Lyme carditis (SILC) score using the COSTAR mnemonic

Variable	Points$^\infty$
Constitutional Symptoms*	2
Outdoor Activity or endemic area	1
Sex Male	1
Tick bite	3
Age less than 50 years	1
Rash- Erythema migrans	4

$^\infty$0–2 points: Low pretest probability of Lyme carditis; 3–6 points: Intermediate pretest probability of Lyme carditis; 7–12 points: High pretest probability of Lyme carditis
*Fever, malaise, arthralgia, dyspnea, myalgia

The Suspect Index in Lyme Carditis (SILC) score is a risk stratification tool, which uses a scoring system to evaluate the likelihood that a patient's high-grade AVB is due to LD [8]. The SILC risk stratification tool was developed following a literature search of English case reports and case series of high-degree AVB in patients with LC [8]. The variables in the SILC score include, (i) constitutional symptoms (fever, malaise, arthralgia and dyspnea), (ii) outdoor activity/endemic area, (iii) male sex, (iv) history of tick bite, (v) age < 50 and (vi) rash consistent with erythema migrans (Table 2) [8]. The variables were developed based on the following findings from the study;

- Constitutional symptoms prior to presentation were commonly reported, which is useful in differentiating LC from other causes of high-degree AV block. Fever was reported in 28.4% of patients and fatigue or malaise in 39.8%. *(2 points)*
- Outdoor activities or time spent in an endemic region were reported in 38.6% and 39.8% respectively, within 30–45 days of presentation with LC. *(1 point)*
- Seventy-five percent of patients were male. This is consistent with a 3:1 male predominance for LC despite an equal prevalence of LD between sexes. *(1 point)*
- Most patients do not recount a history of a tick bite; however, if reported it is highly sensitive for LC. *(3 points)*
- Mean age of LC was found to be 35.8 ± 13.5 years, indicating that LC is an important cause of conduction abnormalities in young, otherwise healthy individuals. *(2 points)*
- The presence of the pathognomonic erythema migrans rash is highly specific for LD, reported in 50% of cases. *(4 points)*

The SILC risk stratification score was tested against the 88 cases identified through their literature review. The sensitivity of the SILC score was 92.3%, in a population of patients previously identified as being positive for LC with 58% having a high SILC score (score 7–12), 35.2% having an intermediate SILC score (score 3–6) and 6.8% having a low SILC score (score 0–2). Specificity was not assessed.

In regard to clinical application, all patients presenting with high-degree AVB should have their SILC score calculated. Patients identified as having moderate or high SILC scores should receive empirical IV antibiotics while Lyme infection is confirmed serologically [9]. As discussed in Chap. 9, temporary-permanent pacing should be considered in those with symptomatic bradycardia. Patients with asymptomatic bradycardia, should have strict cardiac monitoring to ensure that there is no progression of their conduction abnormalities or symptoms. Management of patients with LC following the resolution of their AVB is discussed in further detail in Chap. 8.

4.2   Rheumatic Fever

Rheumatic fever resulting from an abnormal autoimmune response to group A streptococcal infection in a susceptible host remains a serious cause of cardiovascular morbidity and mortality, especially in developing countries [10]. First degree heart block is a minor manifestation of acute rheumatic fever, while more advanced heart block is even rarer. Second- or third-degree atrioventricular blocks in acute rheumatic fever are often transient and self-limiting. Although AVB often resolves within a few days of starting anti-inflammatory therapy, temporary pacing should be considered in patients with symptomatic complete AVB. Rheumatic fever should be kept in mind in the differential diagnosis, especially in pediatric patients with acquired complete AVB.

4.3   Tuberculosis

Tuberculosis caused by *Mycobacterium tuberculosis*, although primarily a lung disease, can affect any organ of the body, including the heart [11]. Although tuberculosis causes various conduction disorders, this manifestation is extremely rare. Especially in endemic areas, when an acquired heart block is detected, it may be necessary to consider tuberculosis in the clinical diagnostic work-up.

4.4   Chagas Disease

Chagas disease, a parasitic disease caused by *Trypanosoma cruzii*, is endemic in Central and South America. Cardiac arrhythmias and transient electrocardiogram abnormalities may be observed during the acute phase of the disease [12]. Cardiac conduction abnormalities may be the first signs, particularly right bundle branch block and left anterior fascicular block [13]. Sudden cardiac death and heart failure are the most common causes of all death. Therefore, ICD implantation treatment should be considered instead of permanent pacemaker implantation in patients with Chagas disease who develop symptomatic AVB [14].

4.5   Infective Endocarditis

Perivalvular extension during the course of infective endocarditis is rare but can lead to complete AVB, particularly when the infection involves the aortic valve. Any conduction disturbances in a patient with infective endocarditis should raise a suspicion towards perivalvular abscess which is a predictor for poor prognosis. Surgical referral is recommended.

5   Infiltrative Diseases

Infiltrative cardiac involvement in diseases such as sarcoidosis, amyloidosis and hemochromatosis may cause AVB's by directly infiltrating the cardiac conduction system.

5.1   Sarcoidosis

Sarcoidosis is a multi-systemic granulomatous disease of unknown etiology, leading to the presence of noncaseating granulomas in various organ systems. Sarcoidosis is primarily a pulmonary disease but up to 30% of patients can present with extrapulmonary sarcoid. Although rare, cardiac involvement can occur in approximately 5% of individuals inflicted with the disease [15]. Complete heart block is the most common abnormality in cardiac sarcoidosis and occurs in 25–30% of patients [16]. It may be the first manifestation of the disease and can occur both in the early and late stages of the disease.

The onset of sarcoidosis most often occurs between the ages of 25 and 60 years of age. Between 16 and 35% of patients younger than 60 years, presenting with complete AVB, have undiagnosed sarcoidosis, which is why it should be on the differential diagnosis in a young patient presenting with AVB even in the absence of other sign and symptoms of the disease. Immunosuppression should be considered in patients with cardiac sarcoidosis if there is evidence of Mobitz II or 3rd degree heart block and/or myocardial inflammation. Permanent device implantation may be beneficial in patients with sarcoidosis who have indications for pacing, even if the AVB is temporary [16]. Pacing is necessary due to involvement of the basal interventricular septum with granulomas and scar tissue. More importantly, the presence of AVB suggests extended cardiac involvement and implies an elevated risk for future life-threatening ventricular arrhythmias. Requirement of cardiac defibrillator should be considered when permanent pacing decision is made [15].

5.2   Amyloidosis

Amyloidosis is a disease characterized by the accumulation of insoluble fibrillar proteins known as amyloid fibrils in various systems. Cardiac involvement is the most important cause of morbidity and mortality in patients with systemic amyloidosis. Although symptomatic conduction system disease is a rare manifestation of cardiac amyloidosis, sudden cardiac death in patients with amyloidosis can occur secondary bradyarrhythmias or ventricular arrhytmias. The prognosis is worse in patients with cardiac conduction disorder due to primary amyloidosis in which the underlying disease cannot be treated [17]. AVB is generally not reversible in these cases and general indications for cardiac pacing and defibrillator implantation should be applied.

5.3   Hemochromatosis

Hemochromatosis is a disease characterized by abnormal iron deposition in parenchymal organs, leading to organ toxicity and dysfunction. Clinical presentation often affects men at a younger age than women, but rarely occur before the age of 40 [18]. Iron deposition may occur in the entire cardiac conduction system, particularly in the atrioventricular node, but can also cause sick sinus syndrome. The presence of this accumulation in the cardiac conduction system can lead to AVB ranging from first degree to complete heart block [19]. Clinicians should consider hereditary hemochromatosis in cases of AVB if there are unexplained liver function test abnormalities, high serum ferritin levels (>300ngmL in men and postmenopausal women or > 200ngmL in premenopausal women) or the presence of an elevated transferrin saturation (>45%). Pacemakers should be inserted for conduction disease leading to symptomatic bradycardia.

6   Autoimmune Disorders

Cardiac conduction disorders are not common in rheumatological conditions but have been reported in cases of rheumatoid arthritis, systemic sclerosis and spondyloarthropathies, such as ankylosing spondylitis. In a Swedish cohort study, ECG abnormalities and cardiac conduction abnormalities were identified in 10% of those with ankylosing spondylitis [20]. It is thought that the conduction disease in those with ankylosing spondylitis is the result of proinflammatory scarring in the myocardial tissue [21]. Conduction system abnormalities have been seen in individuals with extensive cardiac fibrosis from systemic sclerosis [21]. Although these complications are becoming less frequent with the advent of biologic treatment, they should still be considered in individuals with poor control of their rheumatological condition. In young patients, it is also important to consider these diseases on the differential diagnosis for AVB. All patients presenting with unexpected AVB should have a thorough joint and skin examination to look for any signs of undiagnosed autoimmune or rheumatological afflictions that has not yet been diagnosed.

7   Conclusion

Unexpected AVB's are defined as a loss of 1 to 1 AV conduction in an otherwise healthy individual. It can be due to primary cardiac disease or the manifestation of systemic conditions, including inflammatory and infectious diseases; therefore, careful medical history and physical examination is of utmost importance. A high level of suspicion for systemic diseases and a multidisciplinary approach is required to differentiate unexpected causes of AVB.

References

1. Khurshid S, Hoan Choi S, Weng L, Wang EY, Trinquart L, Benjamin EJ, Ellinor PT, Lubitz SA. Frequency of Cardiac rhythm abnormalities in a half million adults. Circ: Arrhythmia Electrophysiol. 2018;11:e006273.
2. Cabrera JÁ, Anderson RH, Porta-Sánchez A, et al. The atrioventricular conduction axis and its implications for permanent pacing. Arrhythmia Electrophysiol Rev. 2021;10(3):181–9.
3. Tracy CM, Epstein AE, Darbar D, et al. 2012 ACCF/AHA/HRS focused update incorporated into the ACCF/AHA/HRS 2008 Guidelines for device-based therapy of cardiac rhythm abnormalities: a report of the American college of cardiology foundation/American heart association task force on practice guidelines and the heart rhythm society. J Am Coll Cardiol. 2013;61(3):e6–75.
4. Van Der Linde MR. Lyme carditis: clinical characteristics of 105 cases. Scand J Infect Dis Suppl [Internet]. 1991;77(77):81–4 [cited 2023 Jan 9]. Available from: https://europepmc.org/article/med/1947815.
5. McAlister HF, Klementowicz PT, Andrews C, Fisher JD, Feld M, Furman S. Lyme carditis: an important cause of reversible heart block. Ann Intern Med. 1989;110(5):339–45.
6. Yeung C, Baranchuk A. Diagnosis and Treatment of lyme carditis: JACC review topic of the week. J Am Coll Cardiol [Internet]. 2019;73(6):717–26 [cited 2022 Oct 8]. Available from: https://pubmed.ncbi.nlm.nih.gov/30765038/.
7. Steere AC, Batsford WP, Weinberg M, et al. Lyme carditis: cardiac abnormalities of Lyme disease. Ann Intern Med 1980;93(1 I):8–16.
8. Besant G, Wan D, Yeung C, et al. Suspicious index in Lyme carditis: systematic review and proposed new risk score. Clin Cardiol [Internet]. 2018;41(12):1611–6 [cited 2023 Jan 9]. Available from: https://onlinelibrary.wiley.com/doi/full/10.1002/clc.23102.
9. Wormser GP, Dattwyler RJ, Shapiro ED et al. The Clinical assessment, treatment, and prevention of lyme disease, human granulocytic anaplasmosis, and babesiosis: clinical practice guidelines by the infectious diseases society of America. Clin Infect Dis [Internet]. 2006;43(9):1089–134 [cited 2023 Jan 9]. Available from: https://academic.oup.com/cid/article/43/9/1089/422463.
10. Holloway AR. Acute rheumatic fever. Pediatr Ann. 2022;51(12):e457–60.
11. López-López JP, Posada-Martínez EL, Saldarriaga C, et al. Tuberculosis and the heart. J Am Heart Assoc [Internet]. 2021;10(7):19435 [cited 2023 Feb 20]. Available from: https://www.ahajournals.org/doi/abs/10.1161/JAHA.120.019435.
12. Miranda-Arboleda AF, Zaidel EJ, Marcus R, et al. Roadblocks in Chagas disease care in endemic and nonendemic countries: Argentina, Colombia, Spain, and the United States.

The NET-Heart project. PLoS Negl Trop Dis [Internet]. 2021;15(12):e0009954 [cited 2023 Feb 20]. Available from: https://journals.plos.org/plosntds/article?id=10.1371/journal.pntd.0009954.

13. Yeung C, Mendoza I, Echeverria LE, Baranchuk A. Chagas' cardiomyopathy and Lyme carditis: lessons learned from two infectious diseases affecting the heart. Trends Cardiovasc Med. 2021;31(4):233–9.

14. Arce M, Van Grieken J, Femenía F, Arrieta M, McIntyre WF, Baranchuk A. Permanent pacing in patients with Chagas' disease. Pacing Clin Electrophysiol [Internet]. 2012;35(12):1494–7 [cited 2023 Feb 20]. Available from: https://onlinelibrary.wiley.com/doi/full/10.1111/pace.12013.

15. Birnie DH, Sauer WH, Bogun F, et al. HRS expert consensus statement on the diagnosis and management of arrhythmias associated with cardiac sarcoidosis. Hear Rhythm [Internet]. 2014;11(7):1305–23 [cited 2022 Oct 8]. Available from: http://www.ncbi.nlm.nih.gov/pubmed/24819193.

16. Birnie DH, Nery PB, Ha AC, Beanlands RSB. Cardiac sarcoidosis. J Am Coll Cardiol. 2016;68(4):411–21.

17. Mathew V, Olson LJ, Gertz MA, Hayes DL. Symptomatic conduction system disease in cardiac amyloidosis. Am J Cardiol [Internet]. 80(11):1491–2 [cited 2023 Feb 20]. Available from: http://www.ajconline.org/article/S0002914997827853/fulltext.

18. Crownover BK, Covey CJ. Hereditary hemochromatosis. Am Fam Physician. 2013;87(3):183.

19. Gulati V, Harikrishnan P, Palaniswamy C, Aronow WS, Jain D, Frishman WH. Cardiac involvement in hemochromatosis. Cardiol Rev [Internet]. 2014;22(2):56–68 [cited 2023 Feb 20]. Available from: https://journals.lww.com/cardiologyinreview/Fulltext/2014/03000/Cardiac_Involvement_in_Hemochromatosis.2.aspx.

20. Forsblad-d'Elia H, Wallberg H, Klingberg E, Carlsten H, Bergfeldt L. Cardiac conduction system abnormalities in ankylosing spondylitis: a cross-sectional study. BMC Musculoskelet Disord 2013;14:237. Published 2013 Aug 12. https://doi.org/10.1186/1471-2474-14-237.

21. Roman MJ, Salmon JE. Cardiovascular manifestations of rheumatological diseases. Circulation. 2007;116:2346–55.

Diagnosis and Management of Lyme Carditis

Kiera Liblik, Mehras Motamed, Cynthia Yeung, Rachel Wamboldt, and Adrian Baranchuk

Abstract

Lyme carditis most commonly manifests as cardiac conduction abnormalities, specifically high-degree atrioventricular block, which may require temporary pacing in conjunction with early intravenous antibiotic therapy. The Suspicious Index in Lyme Carditis (SILC) score has been developed to assess the likelihood that a patient with atrioventricular block has Lyme carditis. Other manifestations of Lyme disease include endocarditis, myocarditis, pericarditis, myopericarditis, pancarditis, and dilated cardiomyopathy. Antibiotics are the mainstay of treatment for Lyme carditis, but cardiovascular dysfunction should be treated according to guidelines for non-lyme disease patients.

Keywords

Lyme carditis • Lyme disease • Atrioventricular block • Dilated cardiomyopathy

K. Liblik (✉) · C. Yeung · R. Wamboldt · A. Baranchuk
Department of Medicine, Kingston Health Science Centre, Queen's University, Kingston General Hospital, Kingston, ON, Canada
e-mail: 14kl3@queensu.ca

C. Yeung
e-mail: cyeung@qmed.ca

R. Wamboldt
e-mail: 17reaw@queensu.ca

A. Baranchuk
e-mail: Adrian.Baranchuk@kingstonhsc.ca

M. Motamed
Department of Medicine, University of Toronto, Toronto, ON, Canada
e-mail: mmotamed@qmed.ca

1　Introduction

Lyme disease (LD) is a tick-borne illness caused by pathogenic species of the *Borrelia* genus, most commonly *Borrelia burgdorferi* (B. *burgdorferi*). In Europe, other genospecies such as B. *afzelli* and B. *garinii* cause significant human disease and are associated with chronic skin infection and neurologic disease, respectively [1]. For further details on the epidemiology of LD, refer to Chap. 2.

The systemic manifestations of LD vary widely and include cardiovascular, neurological, and joint involvement [2]. Lyme carditis (LC) refers to LD manifestations involving the heart. LC most commonly presents as high-degree atrioventricular block (AVB) in 90% of cases [3, 4]. However, endocarditis, myocarditis, pericarditis, myopericarditis, pancarditis, and dilated cardiomyopathy (DCM) have also been reported [5, 6]. Thus, practitioners in regions of high prevalence must be able to detect and treat LC. An overview of the diagnosis and management of LC is presented in this chapter (Table 1). The presentation of LC in the pediatric population is discussed in Chap. 11.

2　Signs and Symptoms

Patients with LC and conduction abnormalities may present with cardiac symptoms including pre-syncope, syncope, and palpitations, but also non-specific findings such as erythema migrans (50%), fatigue (40%), and/or fever (28%). Other patients may be completely asymptomatic. [3, 4] The non-specific nature of these symptoms contributes to the uncertainty when detecting LC (Table 2).

Similarly, patients with myocarditis, pericarditis, myopericarditis, and pancarditis may be asymptomatic or report chest pain, syncope, dyspnea, and other symptoms of cardiac dysfunction [7, 8]. Notably, myopericarditis related to LD in particular can present with symptoms mimicking acute coronary syndrome (ACS) [10].

Lyme endocarditis should be considered for cases of endocarditis in endemic regions with no other identifiable cause, as well as endocarditis in the context of a recently reported tick bite. Signs and symptoms of LD endocarditis are non-specific, and patients may present with increasing fatigue, palpitations, dyspnea, intermittent fevers, anorexia, unproductive cough, or be asymptomatic [6, 9–11].

Emerging literature suggests that DCM may be a rare manifestation of LC, occurring in the late disseminated stage of LD months to years after initial infection. Significantly, severe DCM can progress to heart failure and subsequent transplantation. Patients present with typical symptoms of DCM, such as reduced exercise capacity, dyspnea, and chest pain, although some may be asymptomatic [12].

Table 1 Clinical presentation, diagnosis, and treatment strategies for manifestations of Lyme carditis

Lyme Carditis Manifestation	Clinical Presentation	Diagnosis	Treatment
All Causes *Lyme carditis may be symptomatic*	Erythema migrans Fever Fatigue Malaise Syncope	Enzyme-linked immunosorbent assay Western blot	Doxycycline Intravenous ceftriaxone
Conduction Abnormalities	Palpitations	Electrocardiogram	Pacing Temporary pacemaker Permanent pacemaker
Dilated Cardiomyopathy	Dyspnea Reduced exercise capacity Peripheral edema Chest pain Palpitations Coughing when supine (orthopnea, paroxysmal nocturnal dyspnea)	Real-time polymerase chain reaction of blood or endomyocardial biopsy Electron microscopy	Heart transplantation Standard treatment if heart failure occurs
Endocarditis	Cardiogenic Shock Chest pain Dyspnea Peripheral edema Chills Night sweats	Real-time polymerase chain reaction of blood or endomyocardial biopsy 16S rRNA polymerase chain reaction and sequencing Blood culture Tissue culture Electrocardiogram Echocardiogram Cardiac Computed Tomography Cardiac magnetic resonance	Surgical valve repair Surgical valve replacement Pericardiocentesis if progression to pericardial effusion occurs

(continued)

Table 1 (continued)

Lyme Carditis Manifestation	Clinical Presentation	Diagnosis	Treatment
Myocarditis	Palpitations Chest pain Dyspnea Peripheral edema	Electrocardiogram Echocardiogram Cardiac Computed Tomography Cardiac magnetic resonance	Corticosteroids in refractory disease or if resolution does not occur with antibiotics
Pancarditis	Palpitations Positional dyspnea Chest pain		Pericardiocentesis if progression to pericardial effusion occurs Corticosteroids in refractory disease
Myopericarditis	Palpitations Chest pain Dyspnea		
Pericarditis	Palpitations Pleuritic chest pain Dyspnea Peripheral edema	Electrocardiogram Echocardiogram Cardiac Computed Tomography Cardiac magnetic resonance	

Table 2 Signs and symptoms, electrocardiographic presentation, treatment, and resolution of patients with Lyme carditis presenting with atrioventricular block

	Reported frequency (%)
Signs and Symptoms	
Erythema migrans	50
Fever	28.4
Fatigue/malaise	39.8
Electrocardiographic Presentation	
Third degree atrioventricular block	77.3
Second degree atrioventricular block	33
Asystole/sinus pauses	12.5
Treatment	
Antibiotics	93.2
Pacemaker	44.3
Temporary	71.8
Permanent	17.9
Temporary-Permanent	10.3
Resolution	
Atrioventricular block resolved	94.3

Reproduced with permission, Yeung et al. 2019

3 Diagnosis

3.1 Conduction Abnormalities

The most common conduction abnormality is AVB, which typically occurs in the first two months after LD exposure but may be seen as early as the first week after infection [2]. AVB can develop transiently but when present, can progress rapidly to life-threatening rhythm disturbances. Accordingly, patients are at risk of developing a fatal third-degree block without early antibiotic intervention [13, 14]. The Suspicious Index in Lyme Carditis (SILC) score has been developed to assess the likelihood that a patient presenting with AVB has LC (Chap. 7). Risk factors used in this scoring tool can be remembered with the mnemonic CO-STAR: Constitutional symptoms, Outdoor activity/endemic area, Sex (LC more likely in males), Tick bite, Age, and Rash. Patients are classified as low risk (0–2), intermediate risk (3–6), or high risk (7–12), as demonstrated in Table 3 (sensitivity 93.2%)[3, 4].

Other conduction abnormalities seen in LC include intra-atrial block, supraventricular tachycardia, sinus node disease and dysfunction, ventricular and atrial fibrillation, bundle branch block, and ventricular tachycardia. An electrocardiogram (ECG) should be considered in all patients with LD.

Table 3 The Suspicious Index in Lyme Carditis (SILC) for evaluated the risk of Lyme carditis in patients with atrioventricular block. The variables of interest can be remembered using the acronym "CO-STAR". Based on the score, patients can be classified as having low (0–2), intermediate (3–6), or high (7–12) suspicion of Lyme carditis

Variable	Value
Constitutional symptoms*	2
Outdoor activity/endemic area	1
Sex: Male	1
Tick bite	3
Age < 50 years	1
Rash: Erythema migrans	4

Reproduced with permission, Besant et al. 2018
*fever, malaise, arthralgia, and dyspnea

Myocarditis, Myopericarditis, Pericarditis, and Pancarditis

ECG changes in patients with myocarditis, pericarditis, myopericarditis, and pancarditis may include abnormal left ventricular depolarization and repolarization, manifesting as ST segment and T wave abnormalities. Comparison with a prior baseline ECG is helpful to detect new conduction abnormalities [7, 8]. In up to 60% of LC patients, ST changes and T wave inversion are seen primarily in the inferolateral leads, with rare elevation of serum cardiac biomarkers [7, 8, 15]. Patients with myopericarditis related to LD may have ECG changes mimicking an acute myocardial infarction and elevated cardiac troponin levels [10]. In these patients, a troponin is indicated to assess for myocardial injury. It is also essential that ACS be ruled out with coronary angiography.

When myocarditis and/or pericarditis is suspected, appropriate cardiac imaging should be pursued. A chest x-ray should be used to look for alternative diagnoses and to assess for cardiomegaly. All patients should have an echocardiogram to assess cardiac function parameters such as ejection fraction, pericardial fluid accumulation, and wall motion abnormalities. Diffuse ventricular hypokinesis, associated with decreased ejection fraction, may be seen with myocarditis rather than the regional wall motion abnormalities which are expected in ACS. [5] Cardiac magnetic resonance imaging may help to characterize ventricular functional parameters, wall edema secondary to inflammation (i.e. late gadolinium enhancement), and signs of pericarditis (i.e. pericardial thickening and effusion)[4]. Endomyocardial biopsy (EMB) is the gold-standard for diagnosing myocarditis; however, due to the inherent risks of tissue sampling, EMB is only currently recommended for cases which do not respond to antibiotic management to clarify diagnosis and degree of tissue damage [16].

3.2 Endocarditis

Classic findings of endocarditis include new heart murmur, new valvulopathy on echocardiography, and positive blood cultures [17, 18]. Comorbidities, such as immunosuppression, diabetes and indwelling catheters may increase the risk of contracting endocarditis during LD. [9] Lyme endocarditis has previously been detected in patients with existing structural abnormalities including mitral valve prolapse and regurgitation, bicuspid aortic valve, and tricuspid valve regurgitation [6, 10, 11].

Lyme endocarditis may also occur with accompanying ECG changes, such as AV block [19]. If surgical intervention is required, tissue DNA taken from the valve of interest should be tested with real-time polymerase chain reaction (PCR), as blood and tissue culture may be negative. Limitations of tissue and serological evaluation include the low sensitivity of ELISA in the early stages of LD, persistence of LD seropositivity in resolved infections, susceptibility to cross-reaction with non-LD antibodies, and subjective nature of Western immunoblot assay interpretation. Thus, diagnosis initial should be confirmed with a second test (16S rRNA PCR and sequencing, ELISA, and/or Western blot) [10, 11, 18, 19].

3.3 Dilated Cardiomyopathy

Echocardiography is the mainstay investigation to diagnose DCM once LD has been confirmed. Findings include ventricular dilation and systolic dysfunction characterized by an ejection fraction below 40%. Abnormalities may also be seen on ECG, including indicators of hypertrophy, bundle branch block, left axis deviation, and ventricular dysrhythmias [20]. LC-DCM is further discussed in Chap. 14.

4 Management

Due to a paucity of literature on LC, there are no validated guidelines for management. Typically, temporary pacing and supportive therapy are the mainstays of treatment of patients with symptomatic high-degree AVB. In LC, AVB can spontaneously reverse and treatment predominantly involves the early administration of appropriate antibiotic therapy [4]. Permanent pacemakers are rarely required as most cases of LC resolve with appropriate antibiotic therapy, underscoring the critical importance of early detection and management. Pacemaker insertion has inherent risks, requires lifelong follow-up, and introduces unnecessary cost to the healthcare system [4, 21]. Given the aforementioned, we present a previously published algorithm for the diagnosis and management of LC (Fig. 1) [4].

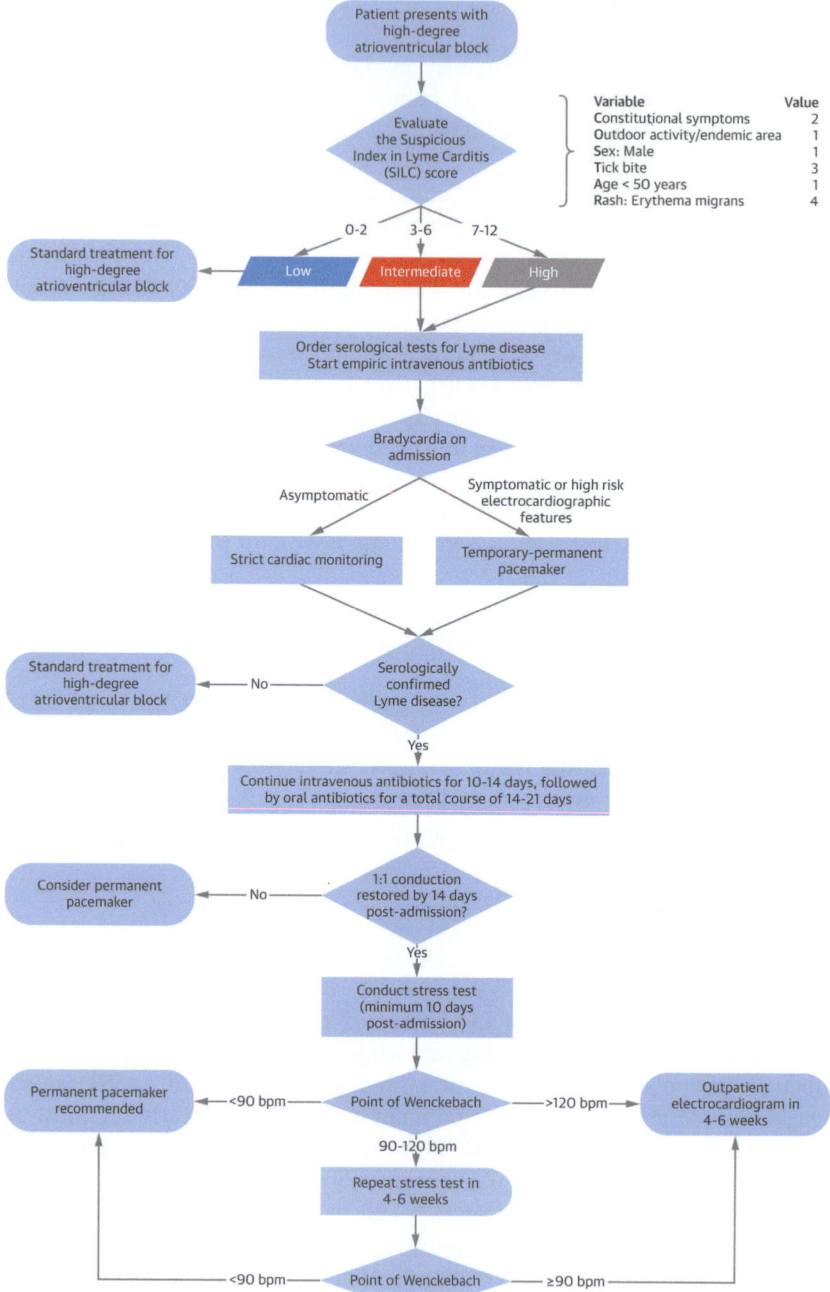
Patient presents with high-degree atrioventricular block
Evaluate the Suspicious Index in Lyme Carditis (SILC) score
Variable
Value
Constitutional symptoms
2
Outdoor activity/endemic area
1
Sex: Male
1
Tick bite
3
Age < 50 years
1
Rash: Erythema migrans
4
0-2
3-6
7-12
Low
Intermediate
High
Standard treatment for high-degree atrioventricular block
Order serological tests for Lyme disease
Start empiric intravenous antibiotics
Bradycardia on admission
Asymptomatic
Symptomatic or high risk electrocardiographic features
Strict cardiac monitoring
Temporary-permanent pacemaker
Standard treatment for high-degree atrioventricular block
No
Serologically confirmed Lyme disease?
Yes
Continue intravenous antibiotics for 10-14 days, followed by oral antibiotics for a total course of 14-21 days
Consider permanent pacemaker
No
1:1 conduction restored by 14 days post-admission?
Yes
Conduct stress test (minimum 10 days post-admission)
Permanent pacemaker recommended
<90 bpm
Point of Wenckebach
>120 bpm
Outpatient electrocardiogram in 4-6 weeks
90-120 bpm
Repeat stress test in 4-6 weeks
<90 bpm
Point of Wenckebach
≥90 bpm

◄**Fig. 1** Systematic approach to the diagnosis and management of Lyme carditis and high-degree atrioventricular block. The Suspicious Index in Lyme Carditis score is evaluated for patients presenting with high-degree atrioventricular block. Patients at intermediate-to-high risk have Lyme disease serological tests sent and are started on empiric intravenous antibiotics. Asymptomatic bradycardia is followed by strict cardiac monitoring, whereas symptomatic bradycardia or high-risk electrocardiographic features (such as alternating bundle branch block) are indications for a temporary-permanent pacemaker. Patients with serologically confirmed Lyme disease continue with 10–14 days of intravenous antibiotics, followed by 4–6 weeks of oral antibiotics. If 1:1 conduction is restored by 14 days post-admission, then the stability of AV conduction is assessed by a stress test. Reproduced with permission, Yeung et al. 2019

4.1 SILC Score and Antibiotic Therapy

Patients with a low SILC score should receive antibiotic therapy upon confirmation of Lyme serology. In cases of intermediate to high SILC score, antibiotic therapy should be initiated immediately, while awaiting Lyme serology results [4]. Most commonly, an intravenous course of ceftriaxone is required until the resolution of acute symptoms and conduction abnormalities (typically 10–14 days), followed by an oral antibiotic, such as doxycycline, on discharge for a total duration of 14–21 days [11, 17, 18]. The use of intravenous amoxicillin and gentamicin for two weeks, followed by a month-long course of oral amoxicillin, has also been effective in a minority of cases [10, 22]. The majority of LC cases will resolve with antibiotic treatment of LD. Antibiotic regimens are summarized in Table 4. For patients with high-degree AVB, within the first 14 days of antibiotic therapy, they typically progress to Wenckebach second-degree block, then to first-degree block, decreasing PR interval, and finally to a normal rhythm (Fig. 2). [4, 5, 23, 24].

Table 4 Antibiotic treatment recommendations for Lyme carditis in adults

Antibiotic	Dose	Duration	
		Serious presentation	Mild presentation
Intravenous			
Ceftriaxone	2 g intravenous once daily	10–14 days (up to 28 days)	-
Oral			
Doxycycline	100 mg oral twice daily	*After intravenous regime,*	14–21 days
Amoxicillin	500 mg oral three times daily		
Cefuroxime axetil	500 mg oral twice daily		

Reproduced with permission, Yeung et al. 2019

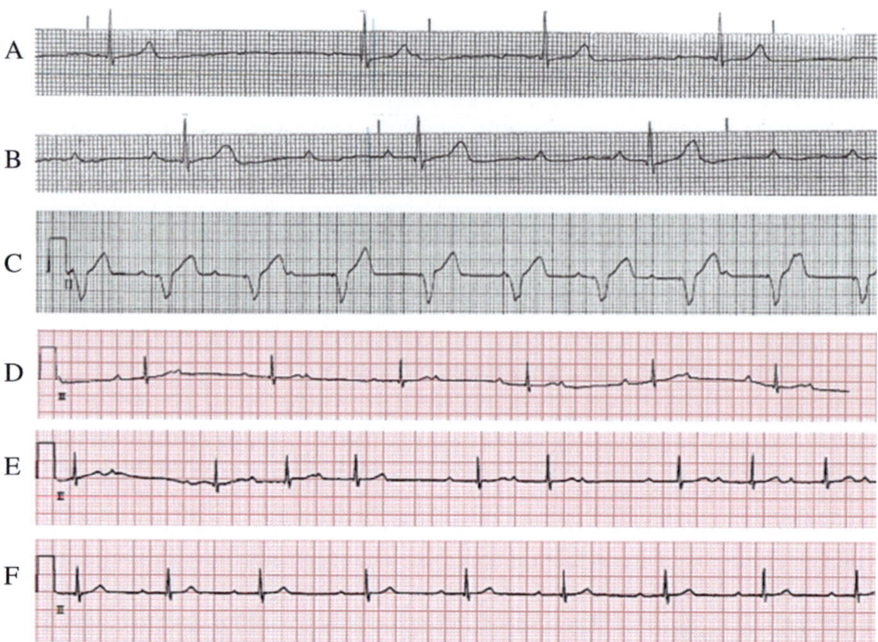

Fig. 2 The electrocardiographic progression of a patient with Lyme carditis presenting with high-degree atrioventricular block (AVB). **a** High-degree AVB (day 1). **b** Third-degree AVB with a junctional escape rhythm (day 1). **c** Temporary transvenous pacemaker placed through the jugular vein due to hemodynamic instability (day 1). **d** 2:1 AVB with a narrow conducted QRS (day 5). **e** Second-degree type I AVB (Wenckebach 4:3 and 3:2; day 7). **f** First-degree AVB with PR interval of 280 ms (day 10). Reproduced with permission, Yeung et al. 2019

4.2 Pacing for High Degree AVB

Temporary pacing is only indicated for patients with symptomatic or high-risk bradycardia. In these cases, standard transvenous temporary or modified temporary-permanent transvenous pacing can be utilized. In order to encourage early ambulation for hospitalized patients with LC, the modified temporary-permanent transvenous pacing device uses an active fixation lead, attached to a re-sterilized permanent pacemaker generator taped to the skin as an external device [4, 5, 25, 26]. Once AV conduction has been restored, an exercise stress test should be conducted to ensure 1:1 AV conduction at a heart rate of > 120 bpm. Permanent pacemaker is only recommended if 1:1 AV conduction is not restored at 14 days after admission. Patients with a point of Wenckebach at > 90 bpm should receive a follow-up ECG four to six weeks post-discharge. If the point of Wenckebach occurs at a heart rate of < 90 beats per minute, permanent pacemaker should be considered. [4] Temporary-permanent pacing in Lyme carditis is discussed further in Chap. 9. If patients undergo implantation of a permanent pacemaker, follow-up with a cardiac device clinic is necessary to screen for restoration of normal AV conduction and consideration of device explanation, which is detailed in Chap. 13.

4.3 Additional Considerations

Generally, the management of patients with complicated LC should follow guidelines for cardiac patients without LD. For example, in case of pericarditis progressing to cardiac tamponade, pericardiocentesis should be performed. Patients with pericarditis should also be treated with anti-inflammatory medications including colchicine and non-steroidal anti-inflammatories drugs (NSAIDs) with careful consideration of additional gastric protection medications. In severe cases of LD endocarditis, surgical valve replacement may be required [11, 19, 27]. Indications for surgical valve replacement are clearly outlined in societal valve guidelines [28, 29]. All patients with LD endocarditis require early involvement of a multidisciplinary team which includes cardiac surgery, infectious disease specialists and allied health professionals. For severe or refractory post-surgical cases of endocarditis, ongoing outpatient intravenous ceftriaxone should be considered and re-operation may be required [6, 11, 30]. Patients with ventricular dysfunction related to myocarditis or dilated cardiomyopathy should be seen by a heart failure specialist for education, optimization of guideline-directed heart failure therapy and monitoring of volume status.

5 Conclusion

Patients living in LD endemic regions are at risk for LC-related morbidity and mortality. The primary presentation of LC is AVB, but several other LC manifestations may impact LD patients, including myocarditis, pericarditis, and endocarditis. LC may also play a role in the development of DCM. Practitioners treating patients from endemic regions with symptomatic LD or cardiovascular symptoms without identifiable etiology should apply the SILC score. Antibiotics are the mainstay of treatment, but cardiovascular dysfunction should be treated according to guidelines for non-LD patients. Early detection and intervention are crucial to prevent long-term cardiovascular damage.

References

1. Kugeler KJ, et al. Estimating the Frequency of lyme disease diagnoses, United States, 2010–2018. Emerg Infect Dis. 2021;27(2):616–9.
2. Shapiro ED, Wormser GP. Lyme disease in 2018: what is new (and what is not). JAMA. 2018;320(7):635–6.
3. Besant G et al. Suspicious index in Lyme Carditis (SILC): systematic review and proposed new risk score. Clin Cardiol. 2018.

4. Yeung C, Baranchuk A. Diagnosis and treatment of Lyme carditis: JACC review topic of the week. J Am Coll Cardiol. 2019;73(6):717–26.

5. McAlister HF, et al. Lyme carditis: an important cause of reversible heart block. Ann Intern Med. 1989;110(5):339–45.

6. Haddad O, et al. Mitral Valve endocarditis: a rare manifestation of Lyme disease. Ann Thorac Surg. 2019;108(2):e85–6.

7. Munk PS, Orn S, Larsen AI. Lyme carditis: persistent local delayed enhancement by cardiac magnetic resonance imaging. Int J Cardiol. 2007;115(3):e108–10.

8. Cox J, Krajden M. Cardiovascular manifestations of Lyme disease. Am Heart J. 1991;122(5):1449–55.

9. Njie AB, Mitchell M, Pukkila-Worley R. Peripherally inserted central catheter-associated nocardia nova endocarditis in a patient receiving intravenous antibiotics for chronic lyme disease. Open Forum Infect Dis. 2021;8(3):ofab041.

10. Hidri N, et al. Lyme endocarditis. Clin Microbiol Infect. 2012;18(12):E531–2.

11. Fatima B, Sohail MR, Schaff HV. Lyme Disease-an unusual cause of a mitral valve endocarditis. Mayo Clin Proc Innov Qual Outcomes. 2018;2(4):398–401.

12. Motamed M et al. Disseminated Lyme disease and dilated cardiomyopathy: a systematic review. Trends Cardiovasc Med. 2022.

13. Centers for Disease C and Prevention. Three sudden cardiac deaths associated with Lyme carditis—United States, November 2012–July 2013. MMWR Morb Mortal Wkly Rep. 2013;62(49):993–6.

14. Muehlenbachs A, et al. Cardiac Tropism of Borrelia burgdorferi: an autopsy study of sudden cardiac death associated with Lyme Carditis. Am J Pathol. 2016;186(5):1195–205.

15. Steere AC, et al. Lyme carditis: cardiac abnormalities of Lyme disease. Ann Intern Med. 1980;93(1):8–16.

16. Radesich C et al. Lyme carditis: from pathophysiology to clinical management. Pathogens. 2022;11(5).

17. Kameda G, et al. Diastolic heart murmur, nocturnal back pain, and lumbar rigidity in a 7-year girl: an unusual manifestation of lyme disease in childhood. Case Rep Pediatr. 2012;2012:976961.

18. Patel LD, Schachne JS. Lyme Carditis: a case involving the conduction system and mitral valve. R I Med J (2013). 2017;100(2):17–20.

19. Canver CC, et al. Possible relationship between degenerative cardiac valvular pathology and lyme disease. Ann Thorac Surg. 2000;70(1):283–5.

20. Bozkurt B, et al. Current diagnostic and treatment strategies for specific dilated cardiomyopathies: a scientific statement from the American heart association. Circulation. 2016;134(23):e579–646.

21. Khalil S, et al. Lyme Carditis in the fast lane: from alternating bundle branch block to Asystole in 12 hours. Conn Med. 2015;79(9):517–20.

22. Nikolic A, et al. Lyme Endocarditis as an emerging infectious disease: a review of the literature. Front Microbiol. 2020;11:278.

23. Krause PJ, Bockenstedt LK. Cardiology patient pages. Lyme disease and the heart. Circulation. 2013;127(7):e451–4.

24. Sangha M, Chu A. Permanent pacemaker avoided in high grade atrioventricular block (abstr). J Am Coll Cardiol. 2018;71(11 Supplement):A363.

25. Fuster LS, Gul EE, Baranchuk A. Electrocardiographic progression of acute Lyme disease. Am J Emerg Med. 2017;35(7):1040 e5–1040 e6.

26. Wang C, et al. Treating Lyme carditis high-degree AV block using a temporary-permanent pacemaker. Ann Noninvasive Electrocardiol. 2019;24(3):e12599.

27. Rudenko N, et al. Detection of Borrelia bissettii in cardiac valve tissue of a patient with endocarditis and aortic valve stenosis in the Czech Republic. J Clin Microbiol. 2008;46(10):3540–3.

28. Writing Committee M, et al. 2020 ACC/AHA Guideline for the management of patients with valvular heart disease: a report of the American college of cardiology/American heart association joint committee on clinical practice guidelines. J Am Coll Cardiol. 2021;77(4):e25–197.

29. Pettersson GB, Hussain ST. Current AATS guidelines on surgical treatment of infective endo-carditis. Ann Cardiothorac Surg. 2019;8(6):630–44.
30. Paim AC, et al. Lyme endocarditis. Am J Med. 2018;131(9):1126–9.

Temporary-Permanent Pacing in Lyme Carditis

Chang Nancy Wang, Sanoj Chacko, and Adrian Baranchuk

Abstract

Most high degree atrioventricular block due to Lyme carditis will resolve with appropriate antibiotic therapy over the course of days to weeks. Lyme carditis patients with atrioventricular block require continuous cardiac monitoring. For patients with Lyme carditis with symptomatic heart block, temporary-permanent pacing is the preferred strategy for ventricular pacing support due to better lead stability allowing earlier patient mobilization.

Keywords

Lyme disease · Lyme carditis · Atrioventricular block · Heart block · Temporary-permanent pacing · Pacemaker

1 Introduction

Lyme carditis (LC) is a rare complication of the *Borrelia burgdorferi* infection affecting approximately 10% of reported cases [1]. Patients may often first present with other features of Lyme disease such as cutaneous, neurologic, and joint manifestations. It is important to consider LC in young patients who present with severe conduction abnormalities, especially if they live in a Lyme-endemic region [2, 3]. Though it can be difficult to diagnose high-degree atrioventricular block (AVB)

C. N. Wang (✉) · S. Chacko · A. Baranchuk
Department of Medicine, Kingston Health Science Centre, Queen's University, Kingston General Hospital, Kingston, ON, Canada
e-mail: chwang@qmed.ca

S. Chacko
e-mail: Sanoj.Chacko@kingstonhsc.ca

A. Baranchuk
e-mail: Adrian.Baranchuk@kingstonhsc.ca

© The Author(s), under exclusive license to Springer Nature Switzerland AG 2023
A. Baranchuk et al. (eds.), *Lyme Carditis*,
https://doi.org/10.1007/978-3-031-41169-4_9

associated with LC, the Suspiciousness Index in Lyme Carditis (SILC) score identifies key risk factors through patient history and physical exam [4]. Since most patients with LC present with high-degree AVB, it is important to recognize this reversible cause to prevent unnecessary permanent pacemaker implantation. Reversal of AVB can occur days to weeks after initiation of appropriate antibiotic therapy [5–7]. Some patients with symptomatic bradycardia may require temporary pacing for hemodynamic support. Traditional temporary transvenous pacemakers require patients to be bed bound, leading to potential deconditioning, and associated increased complications and costs. This chapter discusses the use of temporary-permanent pacemakers (TPPM) for symptomatic bradycardia in patients with LC.

2   Clinical Course of Atrioventricular Block Due to Lyme Carditis

Lyme carditis is usually an early manifestation of Lyme disease but can occur anywhere from < 1 to 28 weeks after initial infection [8]. The most common presentation of Lyme carditis is high-degree AV block, accounting for approximately 90% of cases. Up to one third of patients with AV block due to Lyme carditis may require temporary pacing [9–11]. Other manifestations can include sinus node disease, supraventricular tachycardia, bundle branch block, ventricular tachycardia, myocarditis, pericarditis, endocarditis, as well as valvular disease and cardiogenic shock [8]. The manifestations of early disseminated Lyme carditis are described in detail in Chap. 6.

Most patients with appropriately treated LC have complete recovery within the first few days of antibiotic initiation. High-degree AVB typically resolves within the first 7–10 days but can range from 3 to 42 days [8]. The current recommended approach for patients diagnosed with Lyme carditis and high-degree AVB is to initiate antibiotics as early as possible (sometimes based on a high SILC score while awaiting the results of Lyme serology). Once the patient recovers 1:1 AV node conduction with a PR interval of less than 300 ms, the temporary pacemaker can be removed, and a stress test is recommended to evaluate AV node conduction during exercise. Maintenance of 1:1 AV node conduction at a heart rate > 120 bpm is a positive prognostic sign, and the patient can be discharged home. All patients are recommended to follow-up within 4–6 weeks of discharge to ensure that AV conduction remains within normal limits [3]. On long-term follow-up of more than 12 months after initial diagnosis, most patients have complete resolution of symptoms and conduction abnormalities [11].

3   Temporary-Permanent Pacemakers

Reversible causes of AVB are generally treated with transvenous temporary pacemakers, requiring prolonged bed rest and monitoring in the cardiac care unit due to the risk of lead dislodgement. Immobilization has been associated with complications such as loss of muscle mass and deconditioning, increased risk for venous thrombosis, and prolonged length of stay in hospital [12].

Temporary-permanent pacemakers (TPPM) are "externalized" re-usable permanent pacemakers with an active-fixation lead, allowing for improved lead stability and early mobilization when compared to the standard temporary transvenous pacemaker (TPM). Several studies have found that use of TPPM is associated with decreased rates of lead dislocation and complications (severe bradycardia requiring resuscitation, infection, inappropriate pacing and venous thrombosis) when compared to traditional TPMs [13–15]. TPPMs are an increasingly popular method of pacing in cases where permanent pacemakers are contraindicated, such as in patients with suspected transient conduction abnormalities or active infection.

4   Temporary-Permanent Pacemakers in Lyme Carditis

Patients with LC are often younger and healthier with few comorbidities when compared to the typical population of patients presenting with high-degree AVB [4, 7]. Since the duration of AVB in Lyme carditis can vary and can last for several days after initiation of antibiotic therapy, TPPM offers a stable form of ventricular pacing support while promoting early patient mobilization. At our center in the Lyme endemic region of Southeastern Ontario, Canada, TPPM is the standard therapy for symptomatic bradycardia due to Lyme carditis [16]. Our experience showed that of the 21 patients diagnosed with LC at our center in the last 5 years, 4 patients received TPPM for management of symptomatic bradycardia. The average duration of TPPM implant was 10.5 days (standard deviation 1.9), and there were no procedure related complications.

5   Conclusion

TPPMs are increasingly used for pacing in the setting of patients with reversible conduction or systemic infection, affording better lead stability and allowing for early mobilization when compared to the conventional TPM. In patients with symptomatic heart block due to Lyme carditis, TPPMs are the therapy of choice for supportive management.

References

1. Krause PJ, Bockenstedt LK. Cardiology patient pages. Lyme disease and the heart. Circulation. 2013;127(7):e451–4.
2. Wan D, Baranchuk A. Lyme carditis and atrioventricular block. CMAJ. 2018;190(20):E622–E622.
3. Yeung C, Baranchuk A. Systematic approach to the diagnosis and treatment of Lyme carditis and high-degree atrioventricular block. Healthcare. 2018;6(4):119.
4. Besant G, Wan D, Yeung C, Blakely C, Branscombe P, Suarez-Fuster L, et al. Suspicious index in Lyme carditis: systematic review and proposed new risk score. Clin Cardiol. 2018;41(12):1611–6.
5. Wan D, Blakely C, Branscombe P, Suarez-Fuster L, Glover B, Baranchuk A. Lyme carditis and high-degree atrioventricular block. Am J Cardiol. 2018;121(9):1102–4.
6. McAlister HF, Klementowicz PT, Andrews C, Fisher JD, Feld M, Furman S. Lyme carditis: an important cause of reversible heart block. Ann Intern Med. 1989;110(5):339–45.
7. Fish AE, Pride YB, Pinto DS. Lyme carditis. Infect Dis Clin North Am. 2008;22(2):275–88, vi.
8. Yeung C, Baranchuk A. Diagnosis and treatment of Lyme carditis: JACC review topic of the week. J Am Coll Cardiol. 2019;73(6):717–26.
9. Fuster LS, Gul EE, Baranchuk A. Electrocardiographic progression of acute Lyme disease. Am J Emerg Med. 2017;35(7):1040.e5–1040.e6.
10. Fu M Jianwei, Bhatta L. Lyme carditis: early occurrence and prolonged recovery. J Electrocardiol. 2018;51(3):516–8.
11. Wang C (Nancy), Yeung C, Enriquez A, Chacko S, Hanson S, Redfearn D, et al. Long-term outcomes in treated Lyme carditis. Curr Probl Cardiol. 2022;47(10):100939.
12. Rion JH, Kautz DD. The walk to save: benefits of inpatient cardiac rehabilitation. Medsurg Nurs; Pitman. 2016;25(3):159–62.
13. de Cock CC, Van Campen CMC, In't Veld JA, Visser CA. Utility and safety of prolonged temporary transvenous pacing using an active-fixation lead: comparison with a conventional lead. Pacing Clin Electrophysiol. 2003;26(5):1245–8.
14. Braun MU, Rauwolf T, Bock M, Kappert U, Boscheri A, Schnabel A, et al. Percutaneous lead implantation connected to an external device in stimulation-dependent patients with systemic infection–a prospective and controlled study. Pacing Clin Electrophysiol. 2006;29(8):875–9.
15. Modaff D, Leal M, Kopp D, Teelin T, Eckhardt L, Wright J, et al. Outcomes following implant of semi-permanent pacemaker versus temporary pacemaker. J Am College Cardiol. 2017;69(11_Supplement):426.
16. Wang C, Chacko S, Abdollah H, Baranchuk A. Treating Lyme carditis high-degree AV block using a temporary–permanent pacemaker. Ann Noninvasive Electrocardiol. 2019;24(3):e12599.

Diagnosis and Management of Myocarditis During Lyme Disease

Sebastián Garcia-Zamora, Pablo Iomini, Shyla Gupta, and Oscar Cingolani

Abstract

Lyme disease is a common yet under-diagnosed condition that presents with cardiac manifestations in approximately 1 out of every 10 patients. Although rare, Lyme myocarditis is one of the most serious complications of Lyme disease and can be fatal if not diagnosed and treated promptly. The presence of a tick bite and/or erythema migrans is a "red flag" that should prompt immediate suspicion of Lyme disease. The diagnostic criteria for Lyme myocarditis are similar to other types of myocarditis, but the particular presence of high-grade or complete AV block should raise suspicion for Lyme disease as an etiology. Endomyocardial biopsies are not usually necessary in these scenarios. Early treatment with appropriate antibiotics can change the course of the disease and may even reverse complete AV block.

Keywords

Lyme disease · Lyme carditis · Lyme myocarditis · Atrioventricular block · Heart block

S. Garcia-Zamora (✉)
Italia 1831, CP 2000, Rosario, Argentina
e-mail: sebagz83@gmail.com

P. Iomini
Avenida Presidente Arturo U, Illa, s/n y Marconl Morón 386, B1684 El Palomar, Provincia de Buenos Alres, Argentina

S. Gupta
451 Smyth Rd, Ottawa, ON K1H8M5, Canada

O. Cingolani
733 N Broadway, Baltimore, MD 21205, USA
e-mail: ocingol1@jhmi.edu

1   Introduction

Lyme disease (LD) is an infectious condition caused by bacteria from the Borrelia genus, particularly *Borrelia burgdorferi* and *Borrelia afzelii*. This disease is the most common tick-borne multisystem infection in the Northern Hemisphere, primarily affecting the United States, Canada, and many European countries [1, 2].

Cardiac involvement is typically observed in more than 10% of LD cases. Lyme Carditis (LC) can have a broad spectrum of manifestations, ranging from mild or asymptomatic involvement to severe cases that can result in the death of affected individuals [3]. Therefore, it is essential to consider LD as a potential etiology when diagnosing myocarditis. This is especially important in the early stages, as LC can be cured with targeted antibiotics against Borrelia [3, 4]. The most frequent manifestation of LC is the development of a high-grade atrioventricular block (AVB); however, cases of Lyme myocarditis (LM), including the fulminant form, have also been reported. Hence, in endemic areas, it is crucial to keep this possibility in mind.

2   Clinical Presentation of Myocarditis in Lyme Disease

The term myocarditis implies inflammation of the myocardium, which has many different etiologies, including infectious, post-infectious, drug-induced and autoimmune diseases. Viruses are usually the leading cause of myocarditis worldwide, and the course of the disease tends to be favorable. Bacteria and spirochetes of the Borrelia genus can occasionally cause myocarditis, which are clinically indistinguishable from other etiologies of myocarditis upon presentation.

One of the most challenging aspects of managing patients with myocarditis is diagnosing the disease itself [5, 6]. Many experts have named myocarditis as one of the "chameleons" of cardiology, given its wide spectrum of clinical presentations. The clinical presentation suggestive of acute myocarditis can include:

- *Chest pain*: Acute chest pain, with pericarditic or pseudo-ischaemic characteristics. Chest pain usually starts within 1–4 weeks after an infection, most commonly of respiratory or gastrointestinal origin. Symptoms tends to be recurrent.
- *Heart failure*: New (days to 3 months) or worsening dyspnea at rest or with exercise, and/or fatigue, with or without signs of left and/or right heart failure. Less frequently it can be subacute/chronic (>3 months) worsening of this symptoms.
- *Arrhythmias*: Including palpitations, unexplained arrhythmia symptoms, including dizziness, syncope, and/or aborted sudden cardiac death.
- *Shock*: Unexplained cardiogenic shock, defined as hypotension and organ malperfusion.

Although it is very difficult to make a diagnosis of Borrelia infection based on clinical findings alone, some information from the history and physical examination are "red flags" that should rise the suspicious of the disease [7]:

- Outdoor activity in endemic areas, specifically during summer months.
- Constitutional symptoms: Fever, malaise, arthralgia, and dyspnea
- Tick bite
- Erythema migrans

The last two signs (tick bites and erythema migrans) are highly suggestive of Lyme disease. Each of these signs confers an intermediate risk for patients, so these findings should launch diagnostic investigations (Fig. 1). The Suspicious Index in Lyme Carditis (SILC) score can be used to evaluate the likelihood that a patient's disease is caused by LC [7]. Althought not specifically validated for LM, it an be useful to assess who should be evaluated in more detail. More information is covered in Chap. 7. However, it is important to note that some patients with confirmed LC may not recall a history of tick-bite, which could result in delayed diagnosis [8]. Therefore, it is crucial to maintain a high level of suspicion for LC, especially in patients presenting with unexplained cardiac symptoms in endemic areas.

The most common manifestation of myocarditis is an acute myocardial infarction-like syndrome or acute heart failure [9]. Less frequent presentations include the new onset of supraventricular/ventricular arrhythmias or sudden cardiac death. Lyme myocarditis can also have protean presentations, but its cardinal signs tends to be the presence of high-grade AV block, and even complete AV block [10]. Finally, although rare in the setting of LM, acute myocarditis can be asymptomatic but patients may develop chronic heart failure.

3   Diagnosis of Lyme Myocarditis

The complexity of LM patients cannot be under-stated as currently there is no clear gold standard for the diagnosis of the disease. The initial clues to suspect this diagnosis are an elevation of cardiac troponin (seen in up to 80% of patients with myocarditis), along with new electrocardiographic (ECG) or echocardiographic abnormalities (Table 1). Although these findings are highly sensitive, they show low specificity for the diagnosis of LM.

Traditionally, endomyocardial biopsy (EMB) was considered the "gold standard" for diagnosing myocarditis. However, the patchy involvement of the myocardium raises the possibility that the zone where the specimens are taken during an EMB is normal. Thus, a normal biopsy does not exclude the diagnosis of LM in the context of high suspicion. In recent years, cardiac magnetic resonance (CMR) has gained a prominent place in the diagnostic workup of this disease,

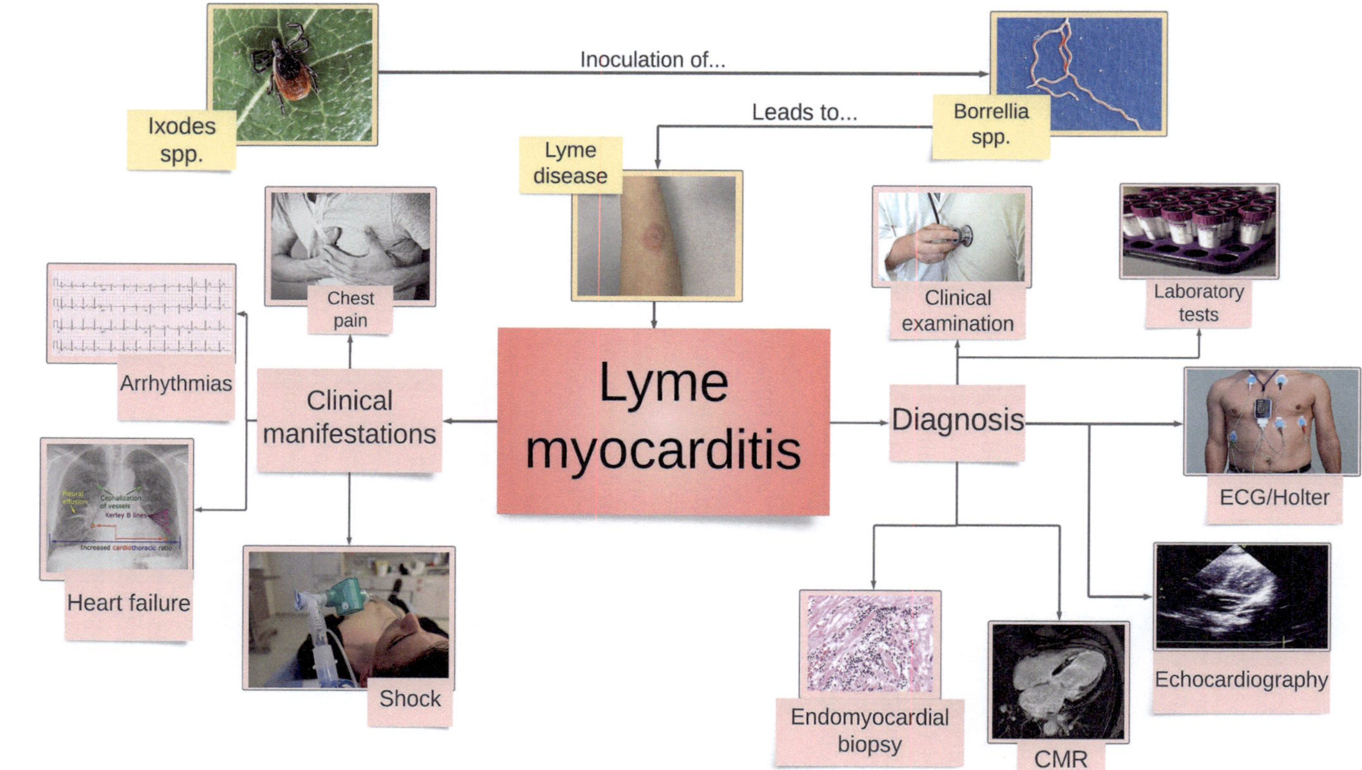

Fig. 1 Signs, symptoms and forms of presentation of myocarditis due to Lyme disease

Table 1 Diagnostic criteria of acute Lyme myocarditis*

Laboratory Testing for Myocarditis
- Elevated troponins (myocardiocytolysis markers) is the more sensitive determination during the acute phase
- Other useful tests that can be considered (depending on suspicion and availability):
- Natriuritic peptides (BNP, NT-proBNP)
- White blood cell count to exclude eosinophilia
- C-reactive protein (CRP) and others acute phase reactants (e.g. erythrocyte sedimentation rate)
- Skeletal muscle enzymes, liver and renal function, thyroid function tests and iron status
- In punctual situations: PCR testing of common cardiotrophic viruses, circulating IgM or IgG antibodies for specific pathogens

Laboratory Testing for Lyme disease
The standard workout is a 2-tiered approach$^\in$:
1. First step: IgM and IgG antibody screening test with the ELISA method (Enzyme-linked immunosorbent assay)
If the results are positive or borderline;
2. Second step: confirmation with Western blot assay

ECG or Holter Monitor for Lyme carditis
There may be numerous alterations, isolated or in combination including; ST deviation, T wave change (T wave inversion or flattening), new bundle branch block, ventricular tachycardia or fibrillation and asystole, 1st to 3rd degree atrioventricular block, sinus arrest, supraventricular tachycardia (including atrial fibrillation), reduced R wave height, intraventricular conduction delay (widened QRS complex), abnormal Q waves, low voltage, frequent premature beats. LC most commonly presents with significant bradycardia secondary to varying degrees of AV block. Progression to high-grade AV block can be very rapid, even occuring within a few hours LM can share many similar electrocardiographic manifestations as other types of myocarditis

Echocardiography
Regional wall motion and/or global systolic or diastolic function abnormalities affecting left ventricle, right ventricle or both. The affected ventricles have varying degrees of dilatation, wall thickness and presence of endocavitary thrombi
Individuals may also present with pericardial effusions

Other Cardiac Imaging
- The most useful test is CMR which allows for tissue characterization, with or without contrast administration. Aside from the findings that can be detected by echocardiography, CMR can show**:
- Edema
- Hyperemia or capillary leak (early gadolinium enhancement)
- Necrosis or scar (late gadolinium enhancement)
- Coronary angiography, or in selected cases Cardiac CT, can be used to rule out significant coronary stenosis
- Cardiac PET can be considered in patients who cannot undergo CMR or with specific aetiologist (e.g.: cardiac sarcoidosis)

(continued)

Table 1 (continued)

Laboratory Testing for Myocarditis
- Elevated troponins (myocardiocytolysis markers) is the more sensitive determination during the acute phase
- Other useful tests that can be considered (depending on suspicion and availability):
- Natriuritic peptides (BNP, NT-proBNP)
- White blood cell count to exclude eosinophilia
- C-reactive protein (CRP) and others acute phase reactants (e.g. erythrocyte sedimentation rate)
- Skeletal muscle enzymes, liver and renal function, thyroid function tests and iron status
- In punctual situations: PCR testing of common cardiotrophic viruses, circulating IgM or IgG antibodies for specific pathogens

Endomyocardial Biopsy (EMB)
EMB is gold standard for the diagnosis of myocarditis, although it is usually reserved for life-threatening cases, when the etiological diagnosis cannot be determined using other tests
At least three to five samples from the right or from the left ventricle should be taken to increase the diagnostic accuracy

Absence of
Coronary artery disease (epicardial vessel coronary stenosis $\geq 50\%$), and other pre-existing cardiovascular disease or extra-cardiac causes that could explain the syndrome (e.g.: valve disease, congenital heart disease, hyperthyroidism, etc.)

CMR = Cardiac Magnetic Resonance; PET = positron emission tomography; CT = computed tomography; ECG = Electrocardiogram
* adapted from reference [5]
** adapted from reference [11]
€ To review the false positive and false positive results of the test, see Chap. 11

given its high sensitivity with a fair specificity [11, 12]. With the advent of the parametric maps (T1 mapping, T2 mapping, T2*, and extracellular volume), CMR has ascended to a place of privilege, as these tools allow for a more quantitative (not only qualitative) assessment. Additionally, CMR does not require the administration of gadolinium, which is a limitation in patients with renal failure [13]. Unfortunately, CMR cannot be considered the gold standard for the diagnosis of myocarditis, for different reasons [14]:

- Although there are abnormalities highly suggestive of myocarditis, they are not all found in all affected individuals and the timeline can be different for each patient. Moreover, the usefulness of CMR is greater during the first days of onset of the disease, but the diagnostic yield decreases after 15 days from the onset of the symptoms.
- It is an expensive study, and it has low accessibility in certain socio-demographic contexts (e.g., rural areas or in low- and middle-incomes countries).
- Some patients cannot be studied with CMR, especially those who are more critical illness (e.g., those with hemodynamic instability or cardiogenic shock, temporary pacemaker requirement, and those with non-MRI compatible prosthetic material).

- Performing CMR is difficult in some contexts, such as atrial fibrillation (especially with high ventricular rates), heart failure, or other comorbidities that limit the performance of apnea, and claustrophobia.
- Finally, CMR accuracy varies with the operator and the center's experience in evaluating suspected myocarditis.

With the aim of simplifying the diagnosis of myocarditis, the European Society of Cardiology published a Position Statement for the diagnosis and management of the disease [5]. For LM, the criteria for diagnosis using cardiac magnetic resonance imaging (CMR) are similar to those for other causes of myocarditis (Table 2). However, caution is required when performing CMR in patients with temporary pacemakers. Thus, when Lyme myocarditis is suspected, the diagnosis is usually based on electrocardiographic and echocardiographic findings, followed by confirmation using serological tests (Table 1). In severe cases requiring pacemaker, it may be prudent to delay CMR imaging for a few days or weeks while the patient receives antibiotic treatment, to reduce the risk of complications. Thus, it is important to realize that the diagnostic accuracy of CMR is greater within four weeks from the onset of symptoms.

As CMR has been increasingly used in the diagnosis of myocarditis, EMB has been relegated to specific cases [5, 6, 15]. While it is important to consider EMB in every patient with suspected acute myocarditis, its use is restricted to situations where:

- There is severe or progressive disease with no response to initial treatment;
- Life-threatening ventricular arrhythmias or high-grade AV block are present with no expected short-term improvement; or
- Specific etiologies are suspected that could benefit from targeted treatment.

Due to the high sensitivity and specificity of diagnostic tests for LD, alongside its excellent response to specific antibiotic treatment, the need for an EMB is exceptional in the course of the disease.

Table 2 The 2018 Lake Louise Criteria for Diagnosing Myocarditis by CMR

Main criteria	*Myocardial edema*: visualized with T2-mapping or T2
	Non-ischemic myocardial injury: detected with late gadolinium enhancement, abnormal T1 mapping or extracellular volume
Supportive criteria	*Pericarditis*: pericardial effusion or abnormal pericardial signal (late gadolinium enhancement, T2 or T1)
	Ventricular dysfunction: regional or global wall motion abnormality affecting the left and/or right ventricle
Lyme myocarditis	Diagnostic criteria are identical; however, in patients requiring *temporary pacemakers*, it is generally recommended to *defer the cardiac MRI* until the patient is stable

In addition to specific investigations for LC, all patients should undergo transthoracic echocardiography to assess the degree of left ventricular dysfunction associated with the infection as well as for the presence of pericardial or valvular involvement. Patients with evidence of significant left ventricular dysfunction will require ongoing medical treatment as directed by heart failure guidelines. Patients may also require long-term follow-up with echocardiography to ensure resolution of left ventricular dysfunction at least three months after initiating therapy.

4 Management of Myocarditis During Lyme Disease

Most cases of myocarditis during LC tend to be mild. However, a small subset of these patients experience a fulminant form, even in childhood [16, 17]. In these scenarios, prompt and accurate treatment can change the evolution of the patients. The approach to patients with myocarditis in the context of LC is essentially the same as any other myocarditis, but with the addition of antibiotic treatment.

Most patients with myocarditis of any etiology with elevation of cardiac enzymes (troponins) require hospitalization for at least 48 h. Typically, myocarditis naturally resolves within 2–4 weeks in up to 50% of cases. About 12.5%-25% of patients may acutely deteriorate or progress to severe heart failure, with a high risk of death of needing heart transplantation. With proper antibiotic treatment, LM has a better prognosis than the general statistics of myocarditis patients. One of the most powerful predictors of worse outcomes in myocarditis is ventricular dysfunction at presentation, of one or both ventricles. The medical treatment can be classified according to the presentation of the patients:

- *Antibiotics*: are the cornerstone in the management of all cases of LC, including myocarditis. For LM, a combination of intravenous and oral treatment is needed, and the length of the treatment varies according to the severity of the disease (Table 3).
- *Arrhythmias*: LM has a higher risk of temporary pacemaker implantation compared to other causes of myocarditis. As the inflammation within the conduction system tends to be transient and resolve over days with appropriate treatment, and most of patients with LM are quite young, it is important to be cautious when implanting a permanent pacemaker. In some cases, a definitive pacemaker can be removed after close monitoring (see Chap. 13) [18].
- *Hemodynamically stable patients* require initial monitoring in hospital for at least a few days, because the risk of worsening or evolving to haemodynamic instability is higher at the onset of the disease. If ventricular dysfunction or heart failure is present, the patient should receive the standard of care for this condition: diuretics according to congestion state, angiotensin-converting enzyme inhibitor (ACE-I) or angiotensin receptor blockade (ARB), beta-adrenergic blockers (with special caution in the context of LC given the high risk of AVB) and mineralocorticoid-receptor antagonists (spironolactone or eplerenone). New treatments for heart failure, such as angiotensin receptor-neprilysin inhibitor

(Sacubitril/Valsartan) or Sodium-glucose co-transporter 2 (SGLT-2), are also recommended in the context of ventricular dysfunction. However, it is important to note that the use of these drugs are not supported by clinical trials in this scenario.

- **Hemodynamically unstable patients** should receive the same interventions that any patient would receive in this context, including intravenous vasopressors or inotropic agents, mechanical ventilation, or ventricular assist devices/extracorporeal membrane oxygenation (ECMO), as a bridge to recovery or heart transplant.
- **Other recommendations**: to date, there is no evidence to use intravenous immunoglobulin or immunosuppressive therapy in Lyme myocarditis.

Based on general recommendations for myocarditis, physical activity should be restricted (in athletes and non athletes people) up to 6 months after the onset of symptoms (Fig. 2).

5 Long Term Follow up

There is a possibility that patients who have suffered from LC may develop dilated cardiomyopathy later on, especially if they are not adequately treated [19, 20]. Although the general consensus in the management of patients with myocarditis is to allow for periodic long-term follow-up after an episode of myocarditis [5, 6], its usefulness in patients with LC is uncertain [3]. In any case, this should be addressed on an individual patient basis by the treating team. Research in this area is ongoing (see Chaps. 14 and 15).

Table 3 Antibiotic treatment for Lyme myocarditis in Adults*

Antibiotic	Dose	Duration	
		Hospitalization	Mild presentation
Intravenous			
Ceftriaxone	2 g, once daily	10–14 days (or up to 28 days)	–
Oral			
Doxycycline	100 mg, twice a day	After intravenous treatment,	14–21 days
Amoxicillin	500 mg, three times a day		
Cefuroxime	500 mg, twice a day		

* adapted from reference [3]

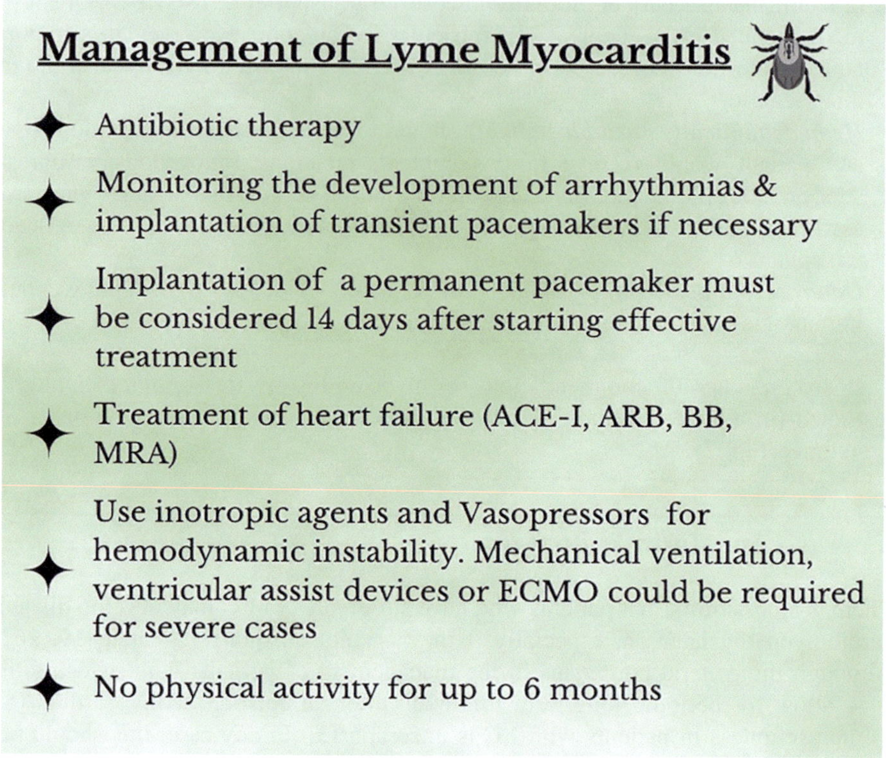

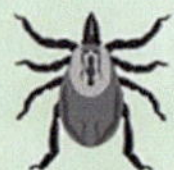

<u>**Management of Lyme Myocarditis**</u>

- Antibiotic therapy

- Monitoring the development of arrhythmias & implantation of transient pacemakers if necessary

- Implantation of a permanent pacemaker must be considered 14 days after starting effective treatment

- Treatment of heart failure (ACE-I, ARB, BB, MRA)

- Use inotropic agents and Vasopressors for hemodynamic instability. Mechanical ventilation, ventricular assist devices or ECMO could be required for severe cases

- No physical activity for up to 6 months

Fig. 2 Main messages in the management of Lyme myocarditis

6 Conclusions

Myocarditis due to LD is a rare but potentially life-threatening condition. A high index of suspicion is needed to diagnose this condition in a timely manner, particularly in endemic zones and amongst travelers who have visited endemic zones in recent weeks. The diagnostic workup for suspected LM should be similar to that of other scenarios of suspected myocarditis. Serological tests have a central role to confirm the disease. Proper and timely antibiotic treatment can change the natural history of LM.

References

1. Shapiro ED, Wormser GP. Lyme disease in 2018: what is new (and what is not). JAMA. 2018;320(7):635–6.
2. Wormser GP, Dattwyler RJ, Shapiro ED, Halperin JJ, Steere AC, Klempner MS, et al. The clinical assessment, treatment, and prevention of lyme disease, human granulocytic anaplasmosis,

and babesiosis: clinical practice guidelines by the infectious diseases society of America. Clin Infect Dis. 2006;43(9):1089–134.

3. Yeung C, Baranchuk A. Diagnosis and treatment of lyme carditis: JACC review topic of the week. J Am Coll Cardiol. 2019;73(6):717–26.

4. Cox J, Krajden M. Cardiovascular manifestations of Lyme disease. Am Heart J. 1991;122(5):1449–55.

5. Caforio AL, Pankuweit S, Arbustini E, Basso C, Gimeno-Blanes J, Felix SB, et al. Current state of knowledge on aetiology, diagnosis, management, and therapy of myocarditis: a position statement of the European society of cardiology working group on myocardial and pericardial diseases. Eur Heart J. 2013;34(33):2636–48, 48a–48d.

6. McDonagh TA, Metra M, Adamo M, Gardner RS, Baumbach A, Bohm M, et al. 2021 ESC guidelines for the diagnosis and treatment of acute and chronic heart failure. Eur Heart J. 2021;42(36):3599–726.

7. Besant G, Wan D, Yeung C, Blakely C, Branscombe P, Suarez-Fuster L, et al. Suspicious index in Lyme carditis: systematic review and proposed new risk score. Clin Cardiol. 2018;41(12):1611–6.

8. Wan D, Blakely C, Branscombe P, Suarez-Fuster L, Glover B, Baranchuk A. Lyme carditis and high-degree atrioventricular block. Am J Cardiol. 2018;121(9):1102–4.

9. Gilson J, Khalighi K, Elmi F, Krishnamurthy M, Talebian A, Toor RS. Lyme disease presenting with facial palsy and myocarditis mimicking myocardial infarction. J Community Hosp Intern Med Perspect. 2017;7(6):363–5.

10. Fuster LS, Gul EE, Baranchuk A. Electrocardiographic progression of acute Lyme disease. Am J Emerg Med. 2017;35(7):1040 e5–e6.

11. Ferreira VM, Schulz-Menger J, Holmvang G, Kramer CM, Carbone I, Sechtem U, et al. Cardiovascular magnetic resonance in nonischemic myocardial inflammation: expert recommendations. J Am Coll Cardiol. 2018;72(24):3158–76.

12. Chareonthaitawee P, Gutberlet M. Clinical utilization of multimodality imaging for myocarditis and cardiac sarcoidosis. Circ Cardiovasc Imaging. 2023;16(1):e014091.

13. Maher B, Murday D, Harden SP. Cardiac MRI of lyme disease myocarditis. Heart. 2012;98(3):264.

14. Grani C. How cardiac magnetic resonance is changing the management of myocarditis. Eur Heart J. 2023;44(11):909–11.

15. Ammirati E, Buono A, Moroni F, Gigli L, Power JR, Ciabatti M, et al. State-of-the-art of endomyocardial biopsy on acute myocarditis and chronic inflammatory cardiomyopathy. Curr Cardiol Rep. 2022;24(5):597–609.

16. Zupan Z, Mijatovic D, Medved I, Kraljic S, Juranic J, Barbalic B, et al. Successful treatment of fulminant Lyme myocarditis with mechanical circulatory support in a young male adult: a case report. Croat Med J. 2017;58(2):185–93.

17. Schroeter MR, Klingel K, Korsten P, Hasenfuss G. Fulminant Lyme myocarditis without any other signs of Lyme disease in a 37-year-old male patient with microscopic polyangiitis-a case report. Eur Heart J Case Rep. 2022;6(3):ytac062.

18. Wamboldt R, Wang CN, Miller JC, Enriquez A, Yeung C, Chacko S, et al. Pacemaker explantation in patients with lyme carditis. JACC Case Rep. 2022;4(10):613–6.

19. Sonnesyn SW, Diehl SC, Johnson RC, Kubo SH, Goodman JL. A prospective study of the seroprevalence of Borrelia burgdorferi infection in patients with severe heart failure. Am J Cardiol. 1995;76(1):97–100.

20. Motamed M, Liblik K, Miranda-Arboleda AF, Wamboldt R, Wang CN, Cingolani O, et al. Disseminated Lyme disease and dilated cardiomyopathy: a systematic review. Trends Cardiovasc Med. 2022.

Lyme Carditis in the Pediatric Population

Cheyenne M. Beach and Jeffrey M. Vinocur

Abstract

The incidence of Lyme carditis is increasing due to the accompanying increase in incidence of Lyme disease. PR prolongation is the most common manifestation of Lyme carditis in children. An appropriate index of suspicion for Lyme disease and Lyme carditis is needed to initiate timely administration of antibiotic therapy. Temporary transvenous pacing is a successful strategy for patients with high-grade AV block and hemodynamic instability. The great majority of pediatric patients have full recovery of conduction abnormalities (and ventricular dysfunction) in the weeks to months following treatment of Lyme carditis.

Keywords

Lyme carditis · Pediatric · Atrioventricular block · Heart block · Lyme disease

1   Introduction

Lyme disease (LD) and its complications are relatively common in endemic areas and in patients who have traveled to these areas during warmer months. Lyme carditis (LC) is one of the more serious complications of LD and requires an appropriate index of suspicion for its prompt and correct diagnosis. The epidemiology, diagnosis, management, and outcomes of LC in pediatric patients will be discussed.

C. M. Beach (✉) · J. M. Vinocur
Yale University School of Medicine, 333 Cedar Street, New Haven, CT 06520, US
e-mail: cheyenne.beach@yale.edu

J. M. Vinocur
e-mail: jeffrey.vinocur@yale.edu

2 Epidemiology of Lyme Disease and Lyme Carditis in Children

LD incidence is uncertain in the absence of mandatory reporting infrastructure but may exceed 300,000 cases/year in the United States (US), perhaps approaching 500,000 cases/year. Among the subset of these cases that are voluntarily entered in the US Centers for Disease Control and Prevention passive reporting system, about 20% occur in children. Pediatric cases of LD and LC follow the same geographic distribution that is seen in the adult population. Pediatric and adult cases of early localized and early disseminated LD also have similar seasonality (typically June through October).

LD affects school-aged children and adolescents at a higher rate than younger children, likely due to differences in exposure between these age groups. LC is reported to occur in about 1–4% of pediatric patients with LD, though numerous sources propose that this is an overestimate as the denominator of children with LD is not known (mild outpatient cases being less likely to be reported than severe cases resulting in hospitalization). The prevalence of carditis among pediatric patients hospitalized with LD in US children's hospitals is around 5%, while carditis has been reported in 16% of those hospitalized with the early disseminated stage of the disease [1]. The prevalence of both LD and LC have increased over time in the pediatric population, with the percentage of LD cases affected by carditis remaining steady, suggesting the increase in numbers of LC cases is due to the increase in cases of LD itself rather than by a change in virulence or cardiac tropism [2]. LC is reported to be less common in Europe than in North America, while pediatric data from Europe and Asia, where LD is also endemic in certain areas, have not been clearly studied.

LD occurs more frequently in males than in females throughout pediatric and adult years. Though the reason for this is not known with certainly, it may relate to different exposure rates. As the risk of developing carditis is related to the risk of having LD, males are also more likely to be diagnosed with LC.

Among pediatric patients with LD, older children are more likely to be diagnosed with carditis. This has been consistently reported, with age over 10 years a risk factor for the development of carditis [1].

3 Clinical Manifestations of Lyme Carditis in Children

Importantly, many patients with objective evidence of LC do not have cardiac symptoms. In one cohort, 50% of children with LD and evidence of LC on an ECG did not report any cardiac symptoms at the time of presentation [3]. If LD is appropriately recognized and treated, these children will likely remain free of cardiac symptoms.

Children and adolescents with LC may exhibit other signs and symptoms of LD at the time of presentation. These may include arthritis, myalgias, fever, rash consistent with erythema migrans, headache, neck stiffness, visual disturbance, and

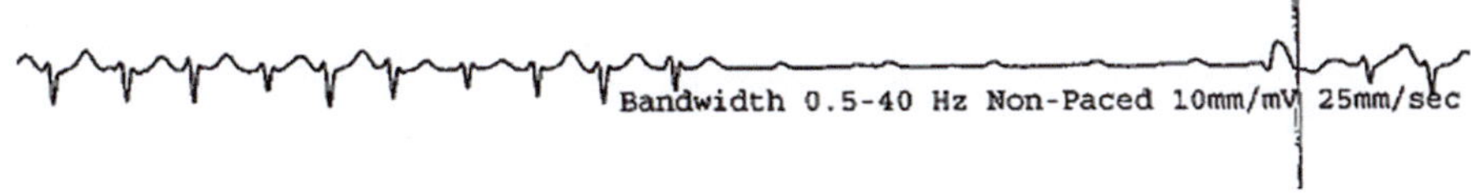

Fig. 1 Ventricular pause in a 17-year-old patient with paroxysmal junctional tachycardia and complete AV block in the setting of LC. There are five non-conducted P waves followed by a ventricular beat and resumption of junctional tachycardia. These pauses are more likely to occur in the setting of increased vagal tone. Reprinted with permission [7]

altered mental status, among others. Lyme meningitis and LC both occur in the early disseminated stage of disease and may therefore co-occur [1, 4].

Atrioventricular block (AVB) is by far the most common manifestation of LC in children. As in adults, conduction system disease is caused by direct invasion of cardiac tissue by the spirochetes that cause LD. A prolonged PR interval (first-degree AV block) is the most common manifestation of LC in children and is seen in about 42% at the time of presentation. Approximately 21% have second-degree AVB, while 5% have complete AVB at the time of presentation [1]. The conduction abnormalities seen in LC may progress rapidly, with complete AVB seen in about 27% of patients at some point during hospitalization [1]. Prolonged ventricular pauses may occur, particularly in the setting of high vagal tone (Fig. 1). Although LC predominantly affects the AV node, often permitting a reasonable junctional escape rhythm, His-Purkinje involvement can occur (reported at 10–20% in adult series and at the case report level in children [5] Fig. 2).

While AV block and associated bradycardia are commonly seen in pediatric patients with LC, other arrhythmias including accelerated junctional rhythm and junctional tachycardia have also been reported [6, 7] (Fig. 1). Other electrocardiogram (ECG) findings in patients with carditis include QT prolongation, ST segment abnormalities, and T wave abnormalities [8]. These repolarization changes are also known to occur in the setting of neurologic abnormalities and in some cases may be related to neurologic manifestations of LD rather than to the presence of carditis.

Pediatric patients with LD can also develop ventricular dysfunction due to myopericarditis. It has been found that 12% of pediatric patients with LC develop ventricular dysfunction [1], with some of these experiencing cardiogenic shock necessitating extracorporeal membrane oxygenation (ECMO) support. In the rare patient undergoing endomyocardial biopsy to assist with diagnosis, "extensive, predominantly lymphocytic infiltrate associated with myocyte damage and necrosis" is seen [1]. Most, but not all, patients with ventricular dysfunction due to LC will also demonstrate AV conduction abnormalities.

Symptoms at the time of presentation with LC are related to the patient's cardiac abnormalities as well as other symptoms caused by the patient's underlying LD. Cardiac symptoms may include lightheadedness, syncope, shortness of breath, palpitations, and chest pain. Severity of symptomatology is related to the

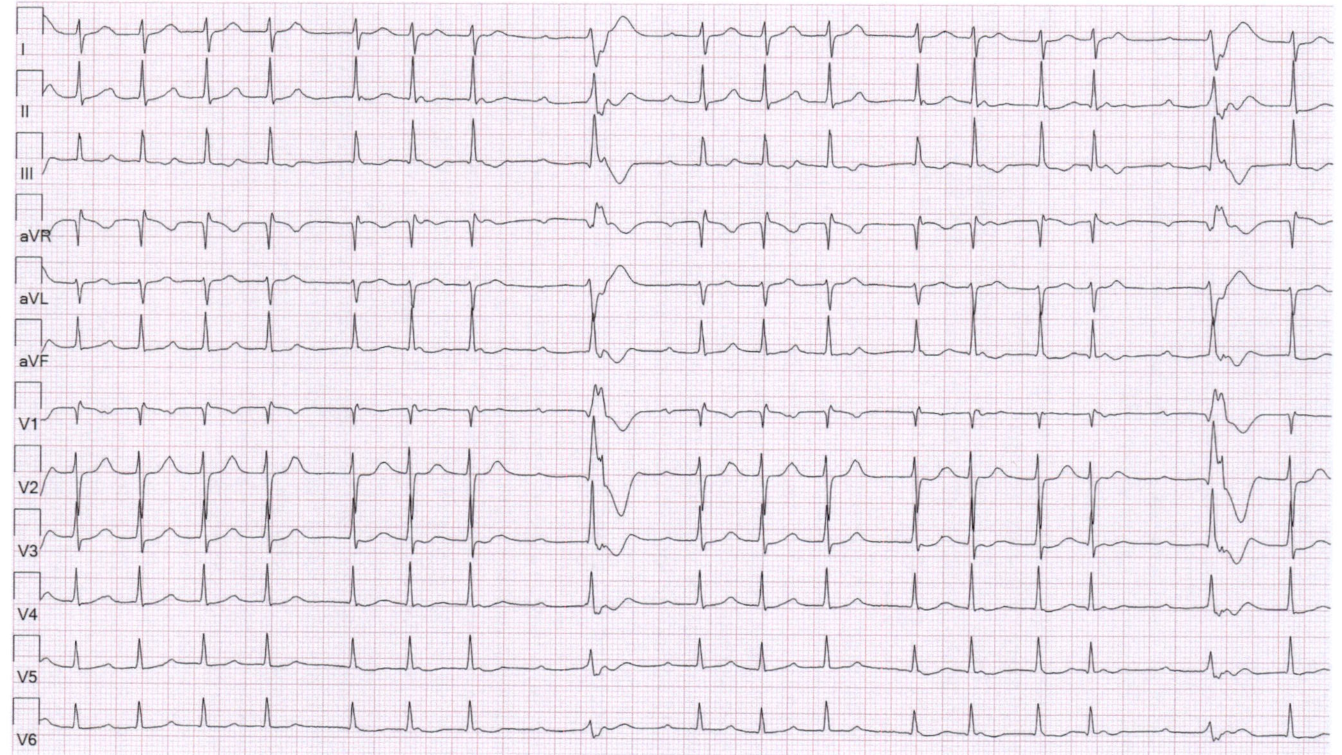

Fig. 2 Erratic AV conduction with left posterior fascicular block and wide-complex beats suggesting phase 4 block of the right bundle or ventricular escape beats in a 14-year-old male with LC who presented with non-exertional syncope two weeks following a viral-like syndrome. Reprinted with permission [5]

degree of AV block, the ventricular rate, and the presence or absence of myopericarditis. Some patients, especially those with relatively mild conduction system involvement resulting in PR prolongation only, may have no cardiac symptoms.

4   Differential Diagnosis of Lyme Carditis in Children

When children present with an ECG finding or arrhythmia suggestive of LC, consideration of the patient's individual risk for tick exposure in a Lyme-endemic area, especially during warmer months, should be made. Recent or current rash consistent with erythema migrans, arthritis, shortness of breath, lightheadedness, palpitations, chest pain, fatigue, and/or neurologic manifestations would increase the suspicion for LD. However, many patients with LC lack a preceding history of tick bite or rash; indeed, these features increase the likelihood of seeking treatment early in the LD course, and so disseminated infection including LC may paradoxically be more likely in those without such clues in the history or physical exam.

Children and adolescents with LC and high-grade AVB typically present with symptoms of bradycardia such as lightheadedness or syncope. Incidentally discovered high-grade AVB without acute symptoms suggests an alternate, chronic diagnosis such as congenital and/or genetic AVB. Notably, patients with distant LD infection may remain antibody seropositive for years, so in endemic areas, patients with non-Lyme causes for AVB will occasionally test positive for Lyme by coincidence.

The behavior of AV conduction at various heart rates can provide insight into the cause of the conduction abnormality. Those with AVB due to LC are expected to have worse AV conduction at higher heart rates; indeed, the first signs of conduction recovery are seen at lower heart rates. In the authors' experience, patients with congenital or genetic causes of AV block tend to have improvement of conduction at higher heart rates. Serial ECGs or use of telemetry and/or Holter monitoring may therefore be very helpful in adjusting a differential diagnosis.

Because LC has particular affinity for the conduction system, it is usually straightforward to distinguish from other causes of myocarditis that tend to have significant ventricular dysfunction and/or tachyarrhythmia by the time heart block is apparent. Selected other pathogens, however, can show LC-like clinical presentation; influenza, for example, has been observed to cause transient AVB as far back as the 1918–1919 pandemic [9].

5   Management and Course of Lyme Carditis in Children

It is imperative to have an appropriate index of suspicion for LD in patients with symptoms suggestive of LC so that they can promptly receive the necessary treatment. It is also important to have an appropriate index of suspicion for LD in patients without carditis to avoid cardiac and other sequelae of the disease.

Patients with early localized LD typically do not need cardiac testing in the absence of cardiopulmonary symptoms, acknowledging that the erythema migrans rash is not exclusive to the early localized stage and can persist into the early disseminated stage. An ECG should be considered for patients with early disseminated LD and is recommended in patients with cardiopulmonary symptoms during any stage of LD. Detailed cardiology evaluation, including echocardiogram, is appropriate for children and adolescents suspected to have LC based on ECG or symptoms. Hospitalization on telemetry is warranted for those with significant first-degree ($\geq$300 ms) or higher-grade AVB, evidence of myocarditis or pericarditis, or concerning cardiopulmonary symptoms, given the risk of progression of conduction system disease and both clinically significant bradyarrhythmias and tachyarrhythmias.

For asymptomatic patients with mild presentations of LC (first-degree AV block and PR interval < 300 ms with no concern for myocarditis or pericarditis), oral antibiotics can be used. Doxycycline (depending on age), amoxicillin, and cefuroxime are commonly used, with specific regimens recommended by the CDC and other groups [10]. Intravenous (IV) antibiotics, typically ceftriaxone, should be used for patients with more severe forms of carditis [10]. In such patients, IV antibiotics should be started as soon as possible without waiting for Lyme testing, which can take days to result at many centers. As improvement can be seen within days, and even hours in some cases, of antibiotic initiation, beginning antibiotic therapy promptly can avert the need for more advanced measures and can reduce hospital length of stay. A typical evolution of AV conduction seen following initiation of antibiotics is shown in Fig. 3.

Placement of a temporary pacemaker should be strongly considered for patients with complete AVB and hemodynamic compromise or evidence of an unreliable escape rhythm. While likely less commonly needed in hospitalized children than in hospitalized adults, temporary pacing is used in up to 20% of pediatric patients hospitalized with LC [11]. Single-chamber ventricular pacing is almost always sufficient; when possible, an active-fixation lead should be placed through an internal jugular or subclavian vein to eliminate the need for bedrest during the recovery process [11]. Pacing is continued until there is an adequate heart rate and hemodynamic stability in the underlying rhythm, most commonly once the patient has recovered some degree of AV conduction. If an externalized permanent generator is used, advanced features such as rate hysteresis can help minimize the pacing burden as conduction begins to return. The duration of temporary pacing in pediatric patients is typically around three to five days [12]. Once AV conduction improves enough to safely remove the pacemaker, it essentially always continues to improve and would not be expected to deteriorate to the point of needing pacing support again.

Avoidance of excessive vagal tone may help to avoid prolonged ventricular pauses. An isoproterenol infusion can be started to increase a patient's ventricular rate, if needed. A dose of 0.02–0.5 mcg/kg/min can be used, with the usual adult range being 2–10 mcg/min. The dose can be titrated to effect, with near immediate onset of action. A good effect is typically seen with doses at the lower end

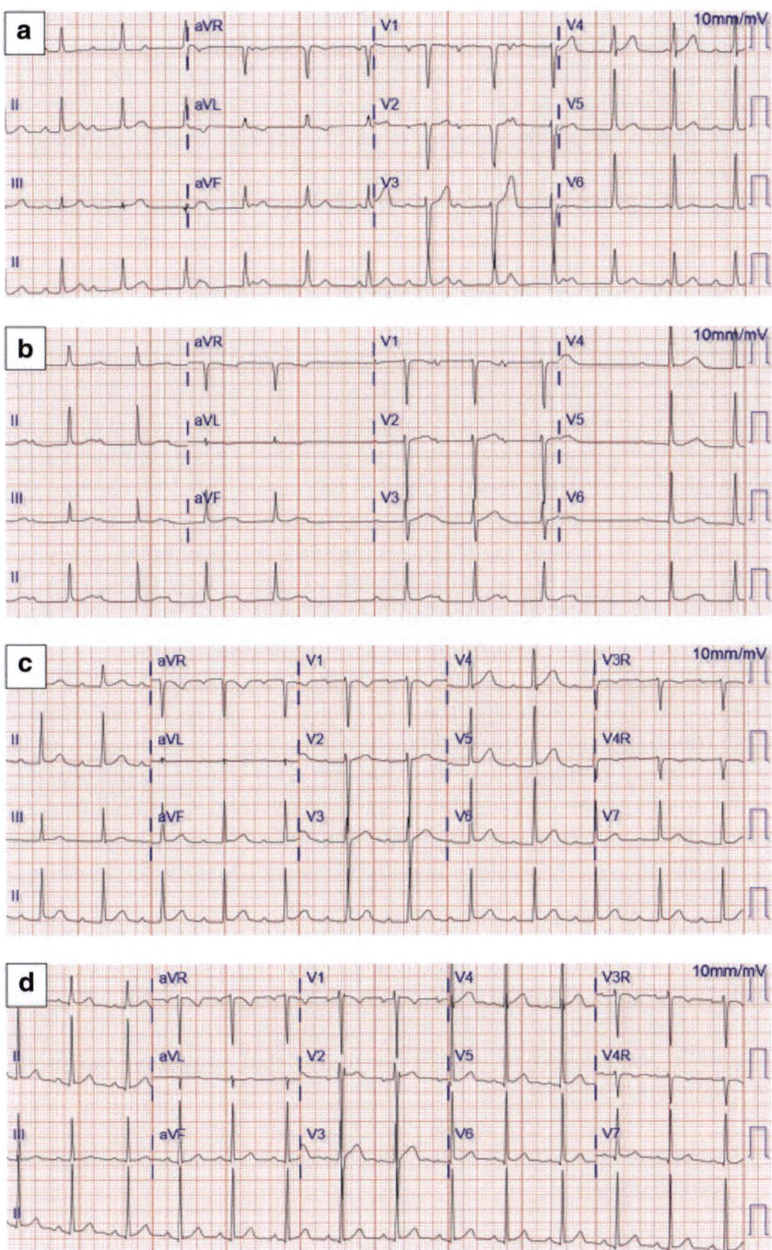

Fig. 3 Typical progression of conduction abnormalities seen in a 12-year-old patient with LC. **a.** ECG at the time of presentation shows sinus rhythm with complete AV block and an accelerated junctional rhythm at 75 bpm. **b.** ECG 2 days after initiation of ceftriaxone shows sinus rhythm with markedly prolonged PR interval of 440 ms and Wenckebach conduction. There has been interval resolution of the accelerated junctional rhythm. **c.** ECG 3 days after initiation of ceftriaxone shows sinus rhythm with prolonged PR interval of 380 ms and 1:1 AV conduction. **d.** ECG 2 months after hospitalization is normal, showing sinus rhythm with a PR interval of 178 ms

of the suggested range, and the high frequency of side effects should be taken into consideration when using this medication. Side effects of chest pain, agitation, restlessness, tremor, nausea, and headache are common and often limit the acceptability of therapy. In the authors' experience, isoproterenol is sometimes used as a bridge to temporary pacemaker placement but is rarely tolerable for prolonged periods. Because of this and concerns about unpredictable tachyphylaxis, temporary pacing is typically instituted within hours of starting isoproterenol.

6   Outcomes of Lyme Carditis in Children

Most patients continue to have some degree of abnormal conduction, typically a prolonged PR interval, at the time of discharge from the hospital. The great majority of pediatric patients have complete normalization of conduction in the weeks to months following treatment, though a small percentage have continued abnormalities. Of the 27 pediatric patients described in one series, 3 (11%) had abnormalities during medium-term follow-up. These abnormalities varied from mild PR prolongation in the initial weeks/months to second-degree AVB up to 2.7 years after treatment [1]. As most pediatric patients with LC are previously healthy, baseline ECGs are rarely available, and it is therefore difficult to be certain that there were not underlying conduction abnormalities in some of these patients.

While some adults require pacemakers at the time of hospital discharge, these patients are more likely than children and adolescents to have underlying cardiac disease contributing to this need. Permanent pacing needs in children with LC have not been described, although it is possible for AVB due to *unrecognized* LC to result in the implantation of a permanent pacemaker for a reversible problem [13]. This unfortunate occurrence can be avoided by maintaining an appropriately high index of suspicion, which includes attention to travel history for those practicing in non-endemic regions.

Deaths in the setting of LC are extremely rare but have been reported. In 2015, Yoon, et al. reported the case of a 17-year-old male who died unexpectedly following a three-week period of viral-like symptoms [14]. A postmortem examination showed diffuse carditis with lymphocyte infiltration, focal interstitial fibrosis, and *B. burgdorferi* in the cardiac tissue and suggested the presence of meningoencephalitis as well.

7   Conclusion

LC occurs in children and adults in similar geographic distributions. School-aged and older children as well as males are more likely to be diagnosed with LD, and, among these, children over 10 years old are more likely to develop LC. A prolonged PR interval is the most common manifestation of LC in children, though higher-grade AVB is seen in a significant number of children as well. An appropriate index of suspicion is required for a timely diagnosis, and antibiotics should be started expeditiously when LD, and especially when LC, is encountered. Temporary transvenous pacing is a relatively common treatment modality during the recovery period, with the great majority of patients experiencing significant improvement of LC within days and resolution of LC within weeks.

References

1. Costello JM, Alexander ME, Greco KM, Perez-Atayde AR, Laussen PC. Lyme carditis in children: presentation, predictive factors, and clinical course. Pediatrics. 2009;123(5):e835–41.
2. Beach CM, Hart SA, Nowalk A, Feingold B, Kurland K, Arora G. Burden of Lyme carditis in United States children's hospitals. Pediatr Cardiol. 2020;41(2):258–64.
3. Neville DN, Alexander ME, Bennett JE, Balamuth F, Garro A, et al. Electrocardiogram as a Lyme disease screening test. J Pediatr. 2021;238:228–232.e1.
4. Kwit NA, Nelson CA, Max R, Mead PS. Risk factors for clinician-diagnosed Lyme arthritis, facial palsy, carditis, and meningitis in patients from high-incidence states. Open Forum Infect Dis. 2017;5(1):ofx254.
5. Maxwell N, Dryer MM, Baranchuk A, Vinocur JM. Phase 4 block of the right bundle branch suggesting His-Purkinje system involvement in Lyme carditis. HeartRhythm Case Rep. 2020;7(2):112–6.
6. Frank DB, Patel AR, Sanchez GR, Shah MJ, Bonney WJ. Junctional tachycardia in a child with Lyme carditis. Pediatr Cardiol. 2011;32(5):689–91.
7. Beach CM, Stewart E, Marcuccio E, Beerman L, Arora G. Lyme carditis presenting as paroxysmal junctional tachycardia and complete atrioventricular block in an adolescent. J Electrocardiol. 2022;4(76):14–6.
8. Woolf PK, Lorsung EM, Edwards KS, Li KI, Kanengiser SJ, et al. Electrocardiographic findings in children with Lyme disease. Pediatr Emerg Care. 1991;7(6):334–6.
9. Cockayne EA. Heart block and bradycardia following influenza. Q J Med. 1919;os-12(48):409–13
10. Centers for Disease Control and Prevention. Lyme carditis. Available at: https://www.cdc.gov/lyme/treatment/lymecarditis.html. Accessed 12 July 2022.
11. Batra AS, Zeltser I. Temporary pacing in children. In: Shah M, Rhodes L, Kaltman J, editors. Cardiac pacing and defibrillation in pediatric and congenital heart disease. Wiley, Incorporated; 2017. p. 195–08.
12. Shen RV, McCarthy CA, Smith RP. Lyme carditis in hospitalized children and adults, a case series. Open Forum Infect Dis 2021;8(7):ofab140.
13. Wamboldt R, Wang CN, Miller JC, Enriquez A, Yeung C, et al. Pacemaker explantation in patients with Lyme carditis. J Am Coll Cardiol Case Rep. 2022;4(10):613–6.
14. Yoon EC, Vail E, Kleinman G, Lento PA, Li S, Wang G, et al. Lyme disease: a case report of a 17-year-old male with fatal Lyme carditis. Cardiovasc Pathol 2015;24(5):317–21.

Early Disseminated Lyme Carditis: Long-Term Follow-Up

Chang Nancy Wang, Reem Al Rawi, and Adrian Baranchuk

Abstract

Lyme carditis commonly presents with high degree atrioventricular block, but most conduction abnormalities will resolve with appropriate antibiotic therapy. Most patients with treated Lyme carditis remain symptom-free without lasting or recurrent conduction abnormalities in long term follow-up of greater than 12 months after initial presentation.

Keywords

Long-term follow-up · Lyme carditis · Lyme disease · Heart block · Atrioventricular block

1 Introduction

Lyme disease is a tick-born bacterial infection caused by *Borrelia burgdorferi*. It is the most reported vector-born disease in North America, and its incidence has risen dramatically in recent years. In up to 10% of cases, dissemination of LD may lead to cardiac tissue inflammation and Lyme carditis (LC) [1]. The most common presentation of LC is high-degree atrioventricular block (AVB) which can fluctuate rapidly over minutes, hours, or days. Most AVB in LC resolve with appropriate antibiotic treatment without requirement of a permanent pacemaker [1–3].

C. N. Wang (✉) · A. Baranchuk
Department of Medicine, Kingston Health Sciences Centre, Queen's University, Kingston, Canada
e-mail: chwang@qmed.ca

A. Baranchuk
e-mail: Adrian.Baranchuk@kingstonhsc.ca

R. Al Rawi
Queen's University, Kingston, ON, Canada
e-mail: reem.alrawi@queensu.ca

© The Author(s), under exclusive license to Springer Nature Switzerland AG 2023
A. Baranchuk et al. (eds.), *Lyme Carditis*,
https://doi.org/10.1007/978-3-031-41169-4_12

The diagnosis and management of early disseminated LC is now well-established, with the use of the SILC (Suspicious Index in Lyme Carditis) score to assess for risk of LC in patients presenting with AVB [2], hospitalization with appropriate cardiac monitoring, targeted antibiotic therapy, and treadmill ECG stress testing to assess atrioventricular conduction stability prior to discharge [3]. Temporary pacing with an endocardial lead connected to an external permanent pacemaker allows early patient mobility for those with symptomatic bradycardia [4]. Follow-up of patients who do not require permanent pacing at 4–6 weeks after initial discharge is recommended to ensure resolution of conduction abnormalities [1]. However, studies on the long-term outcomes of treated LC are scarce, and there is currently no clinical precedence for ongoing monitoring of patients after discharge from hospital.

2   Appropriate Treatment of Lyme Carditis

The diagnosis and management of LC is explored in detail in Chap. 8. In brief, patients presenting with high degree atrioventricular block should be assessed for risk of LC using the SILC score, and all patients should be hospitalized with continuous cardiac monitoring. Those determined to be high risk for LC should have empiric intravenous antibiotic therapy initiated while waiting for serology. Appropriate antibiotic regimens include intravenous antibiotics for 10–14 days (ceftriaxone is first line) followed by oral antibiotics (doxycycline, amoxicillin, cefuroxime) to complete a 14–21 day course [1, 5].

3   Long-Term Follow-Up of Lyme Carditis—Existing Literature

To better gauge the documentation and length of long-term follow up of LC patients after receiving antibiotic treatment in current literature, we performed an informal systematic review. The review was completed on September 28, 2022 using the databases Embase and Medline. The search terms utilized were inspired by a systematic review completed on October 3, 2017 of all published cases of LC with high-degree AVB [2]. Specifically, the search term used was as follows: ("Lyme" OR "Lyme disease") AND ("carditis," "myocarditis," "heart block," "heart muscle conduction disturbance," "heart conduction system," "sick sinus syndrome," "heart arrest," "conduction," "AV block," "atrioventricular block," "asystole," "sinus pause," OR "bundle branch block")). All papers with greater than 1 month follow-up of patients with confirmed LC, published in the English language were reviewed independently by authors C. Wang and R. Al Rawi.

A total of 19 articles were retrieved from the review, giving 31 patients; results are summarised in Table 1 and Fig. 1. Fourteen (73.7%) articles documented only 1 patient, one (5.26%) documented 2 patients, one (5.26%) documented 3 patients, two (10.5%) documented 4 patients, and one (5.26%) documented 6 patients. The mean length of long-term follow up was 8.70 months. Of the patients who received appropriate therapy for early disseminated Lyme disease, all had complete resolution of symptoms and conduction abnormalities. However, the diagnosis of Lyme disease was often delayed, and seven patients received insertion of a permanent pacemaker before diagnosis of LC was made. In four cases, subsequent follow-up also revealed resolution of symptoms and conduction abnormalities. Three patients showed persistence of complete AV block 7 weeks with pacemaker dependency, though this was after sub-optimal IV antibiotic treatment [6–8].

4 Long-Term Follow-Up of Lyme Carditis—New Insights

Recognizing the absence of high-quality data on the long-term follow-up of patients with treated LC, Wang et al. published a prospective single center series on the outcomes of patient diagnosed with LC who received appropriate antibiotic therapy without permanent pacing for high-degree AVB [9]. All patients were asymptomatic and free of conduction abnormalities at a mean follow-up of 20 months with no residual defects.

This new data in addition to existing literature on management of LC supports avoidance of permanent pacing and the associated long-term consequences if conduction is stable at discharge. It is possible that adequate antibiotic therapy may resolve inflammation of the conduction system [10, 11], both normalizing and preserving conduction during long-term follow-up. Since patients presenting with LC are often young and otherwise healthy [1], avoiding unnecessary pacemaker implantation is of the utmost importance to avoid exposure to pacemaker-related complications and long-term consequences [12]. Chapter 13 explores the safe explantation of permanent pacemakers in patients subsequently diagnosed with and appropriately treated for LC.

5 Conclusions

Though data on the long-term follow-up outcomes of patients with treated LC are largely limited to case reports and case series, all available literature supports the avoidance of permanent pacing in appropriately treated early disseminated LC if AV node conduction is stable at discharge. Further prospective studies are necessary to develop evidence-based guidelines for the long-term management of patients with treated LC.

Table 1 Previous literature on follow-up of treated Lyme carditis (>1 month)

Paper	# of Pts	Pacemaker Placed (TPM or PPM)	Adequate abx treatment (Y/N)	Average Length of Follow-up	Symptomatic or Asymptomatic at Follow-up
Isath, A 2018 (6)	1	TPM then leadless PPM	N	1 year	Asymptomatic
Sangha [7]	1	N/A	Y	30 days	Asymptomatic
Afari [8]	1	N/A	Y	1 month	Asymptomatic
Brownstein [9]	1	PPM	Y	3 months	Asymptomatic
Oktay [10]	1	N/A	Y	7 weeks	Asymptomatic
Mannava [11]	1	N/A	Y	2 months	Asymptomatic
Shenthar [12]	1	N/A	Y	2 months	Asymptomatic
Brunner [13]	1	N/A	Y	1 month	Asymptomatic
Wong [14]	1	PPM	Y	1 month	Asymptomatic
Silver [15]	2	N/A	Y	9.5 months	Asymptomatic
Seslar [16]	3	N/A	Y	24 months, 2 patients loss to follow-up	Asymptomatic
Rosenfeld [17]	1	PPM	N	3 months	Asymptomatic
Midttun [18]	6	33% TPM	66% Y	3.84 years	Asymptomatic
Artigao [19]	1	PPM	N	1 year	Symptomatic*
Van der Linde [20]	4	25% TPM, 25% PPM	25% Y	7.25 weeks	25% symptomatic*
McAlister [21]	4	75% TPM, 25% PPM	25% Y	18.75 months	25% symptomatic*
Lorincz [22]	1	TPM	N	18 months	Asymptomatic
Kimball [23]	1	N/A	N	6 weeks	Asymptomatic
Bedell [24]	1	N/A	N	6 months	Asymptomatic

Abbreviations pt = patient, TPM = temporary pacemaker, PPM = temporary permanent pacemaker

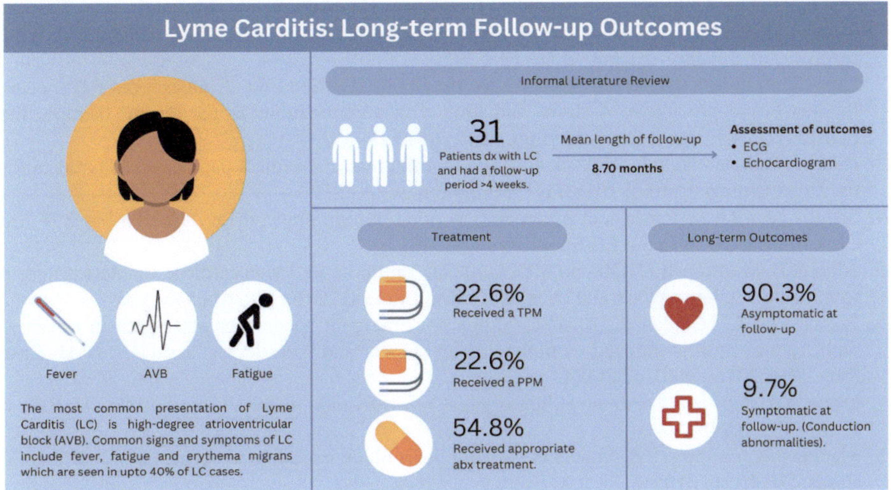

Fig. 1 Summary of existing literature on the long-term follow-up of Lyme carditis (> 4 weeks). *Created Using Canva. Abbreviations: *AVB* = atrioventricular block; *ECG* = electrocardiogram; *LC* = Lyme carditis; *PPM* = permanent pacemaker; TPM = temporary permanent pacemaker

References

1. Yeung C, Baranchuk A. Diagnosis and treatment of lyme carditis: JACC review topic of the week. J Am Coll Cardiol. 2019;73(6):717–26.
2. Besant G, Wan D, Yeung C, Blakely C, Branscombe P, Suarez-Fuster L, et al. Suspicious index in Lyme carditis: systematic review and proposed new risk score. Clin Cardiol. 2018;41(12):1611–6.
3. Yeung C, Baranchuk A. Systematic approach to the diagnosis and treatment of lyme carditis and high-degree atrioventricular block. Healthcare. 2018;6(4):119.
4. Wang C, Chacko S, Abdollah H, Baranchuk A. Treating Lyme carditis high-degree AV block using a temporary–permanent pacemaker. Ann Noninvasive Electrocardiol. 2019;24(3):e12599.
5. Stanek G, Wormser GP, Gray J, Strle F. Lyme borreliosis. The Lancet. 2012;379(9814):461–73.
6. van der Linde MR, Crijns HJ, de Koning J, Hoogkamp-Korstanje JA, de Graaf JJ, Piers DA, et al. Range of atrioventricular conduction disturbances in Lyme borreliosis: a report of four cases and review of other published reports. Heart. 1990;63(3):162–8.
7. Artigao R, Torres G, Guerrero A, Jimenez-Mena M, Paredes MB. Irreversible complete heart block in lyme disease. Am J Med. 1991;90(4):531–3.
8. McAlister HF, Klementowicz PT, Andrews C, Fisher JD, Feld M, Furman S. Lyme Carditis: an important cause of reversible heart block. Ann Intern Med. 1989;110(5):339–45.
9. Wang C (Nancy), Yeung C, Enriquez A, Chacko S, Hanson S, Redfearn D, et al. Long-term outcomes in treated Lyme carditis. Curr Probl Cardiol. 2022;47(10):100939.
10. Olson CM, Bates TC, Izadi H, Radolf JD, Huber SA, Boyson JE, et al. Local production of IFN-γ by invariant NKT cells modulates acute lyme carditis. J Immunol. 2009;182(6):3728–34.

11. Muehlenbachs A, Bollweg BC, Schulz TJ, Forrester JD, DeLeon CM, Molins C, et al. Cardiac tropism of borrelia burgdorferi: an autopsy study of sudden cardiac death associated with lyme carditis. Am J Pathol. 2016;186(5):1195–205.

12. Udo EO, Zuithoff NPA, van Hemel NM, de Cock CC, Hendriks T, Doevendans PA, et al. Incidence and predictors of short- and long-term complications in pacemaker therapy: the FOLLOWPACE study. Heart Rhythm. 2012;9(5):728–35.

13. Isath A, Padmanabhan D, Naksuk N, Kella D, Friedman P. Leadless pacemaker in lyme carditis. J Am College Cardiol 2018;71(11, Supplement):A2531

14. Sangha M, Chu A. Permanent pacemaker avoided in high grade atrioventricular block. J Am College Cardiol. 2018;71(11, Supplement):A363.

15. Afari ME, Marmoush F, Rehman MU, Gorsi U, Yammine JF. Lyme carditis: an interesting trip to third-degree heart block and back. Case Rep Cardiol. 2016;6(2016):e5454160.

16. Brownstein AJ, Gautam S, Bhatt P, Nanna M. Emergent pacemaker placement in a patient with Lyme carditis-induced complete heart block and ventricular asystole. BMJ Case Rep. 2016;2016:bcr2016214474.

17. Oktay AA, Dibs SR, Friedman H. Sinus pause in association with lyme carditis. Tex Heart Inst J. 2015;42(3):248–50.

18. Mannava K, Grabinski Z, Mousa O. Putting heart block back in the "Lyme Light". J Cardiol Cases. 2014;11(4):105–8.

19. Shenthar J, Shetty SB, Krishnamurthy D. Diagnosis not to be missed: lyme carditis, rare but reversible cause of complete atrioventricular block. Indian Heart J. 2014;66(6):723–6.

20. Brunner FJ, Blankenberg S, Sydow K. Digital camera revealed infection with Borrelia burgdorferi as a cause of reversible total AV block in a 42year old man. Int J Cardiol. 2014;177(3):e165–6.

21. Wong DW, Apostolidou E, Bruno C. Lyme carditis presenting with complete heart block in a patient who received a heart transplant. Infect Dis Clin Pract. 2013;21(5):e30.

22. Silver E, Pass RH, Kaufman S, Hordof AJ, Liberman L. Complete heart block due to lyme carditis in two pediatric patients and a review of the literature. Congenit Heart Dis. 2007;2(5):338–41.

23. Seslar SP, Berul CI, Burklow TR, Cecchin F, Alexander ME. Transient prolonged corrected QT interval in lyme disease. J Pediatr. 2006;148(5):692–7.

24. Rosenfeld ME, Beckerman B, Ward MF, Sama A. Lyme carditis: complete AV dissociation with episodic asystole presenting as syncope in the emergency department. J Emerg Med. 1999;17(4):661–4.

25. Midttun M, Lebech AM, Hansen K, Videbaek J. Lyme carditis: a clinical presentation and long time follow-up. Scand J Infect Dis. 1997;29(2):153–7.

26. Lórincz I, Lakos A, Kovács P, Várvölgyi C, Polgár P, Wórum F. Temporary pacing in complete heart block due to Lyme disease: a case report. Pacing Clin Electrophysiol. 1989;12(8):1433–6.

27. Kimball SA, Janson PA, LaRaia PJ. Complete heart block as the sole presentation of lyme disease. Arch Intern Med. 1989;149(8):1897–8.

28. Bedell SE, Pastor BM, Cohen SI. Symptomatic high grade heart block in lyme disease. Chest. 1981;79(2):236–7.

Considerations for Permanent Pacemaker Explantation in Resolved Lyme Carditis

Rachel Wamboldt, Sanoj Chacko, and Adrian Baranchuk

Abstract

Permanent pacemakers should not be part of the treatment algorithm for Lyme carditis (LC), as LC is a transient cause of high-degree atrioventricular (AV) block that should resolve after 5–10 days of intravenous antibiotics. If LC is not suspected by the treating physicians, the patient may undergo the unnecessary implantation of a permanent pacemaker. If the diagnosis of LC is confirmed after permanent pacemaker implantation, the pacemaker may be safely explanted within the first year as long as the patient has completed a three-week course of antibiotics, no evidence of ventricular pacing on interrogation, and a stress-test confirming 1:1 AV conduction during exercise.

Keywords

Lyme carditis • Lyme disease • Pacemaker explantation • Heart block • Atrioventricular block

1 Introduction

Lyme carditis (LC) is a clinical manifestation of early disseminated Lyme disease (LD) that results in alterations in cardiac function, particularly the conduction system. Patients with any evidence of LC should be admitted to the hospital for monitoring and intravenous antibiotics. If symptomatic bradycardia occurs from

R. Wamboldt (✉) · S. Chacko · A. Baranchuk
76 Stuart Street, Kingston, Ontario K7L 3N6, Canada
e-mail: 17reaw@queensu.ca

S. Chacko
e-mail: Sanoj.Chacko@kingstonhsc.ca

A. Baranchuk
e-mail: Adrian.Baranchuk@kingstonhsc.ca

either a high-grade AV nodal conduction disturbance or sinus node dysfunction, patients may require treatment with a temporary pacing device to support their cardiac rhythm while their conduction system recovers [1, 2]. Permanent pacemakers should not be a part of the treatment algorithm for LC, unless in the exceedingly rare circumstance that their conduction abnormality does not recover following a course of guideline-directed antibiotics [1, 3].

The diagnosis of LC is made predominantly from clinical presentation, with confirmatory serological testing [1]. Unfortunately, making the diagnosis of LC can be challenging and requires a high degree of clinical suspicion, given that it typically manifests 1–2 months after the initial infection with *Borrelia burgdorferi*. [4] If LD is not considered within the differential diagnosis for symptomatic bradycardia or if physicians do not allow adequate time for conduction system recovery, following the administration of antibiotics, patients may undergo the unnecessary placement of a permanent pacing device. In such cases, if these patients are identified early, and their cardiac rhythm recovers following antibiotics, pacemaker explantation should be facilitated. Before device explanation is arranged, several considerations are required. This chapter will outline the risks associated with inappropriate pacemaker implantation and how device explantation can be facilitated safely.

2   Pacemakers in Lyme Carditis

The insertion of a permanent pacing device is an invasive procedure. Complications related to the procedure are rare but can be serious (Table 1) [5, 6] Given the young age of patients with LC, the unnecessary implantation of a permanent pacemaker can also lead to a lifetime of physical and psychological consequences, frequent device checks, and an accumulation of health care costs [1]. In the event that a patient has had a permanent pacing device implanted as part of their treatment for LC, regular follow-up with a cardiac device clinic is necessary to ensure that the pacemaker is functioning appropriately, to screen for complications and to assess for ventricular pacing. Once there is convincing evidence of complete recovery of the conduction system with resolution of ventricular pacing, pacemaker and lead explantation should be facilitated (Fig. 1). [2] If performed within the first year of implantation, lead explantation can be performed using simple traction techniques, using regular stylets [5]. Traction techniques in these cases have a high success rate with a low risk of complications [5].

Chronically implanted pacemaker leads (> 1-year duration) can develop fibrotic attachments at the tip of the wire as well as throughout its length [5, 6]. The presence of fibrotic attachments to the veins (access vein or superior vena cava) and endocardial structures (valves, papillary muscles, endocardium, electrode-myocardial interface), increase the risk of complications associated with lead removal [5]. Separating the lead from the encapsulating tissue is the most crucial step in the process of lead extraction. The lead extraction procedure can be performed using a variety of techniques including traction (simple, continuous),

Table 1 Procedural, short-term, and long-term complications associated with pacemaker insertion for Lyme carditis

Procedural complications	Short-term complications	Long-term complications
- Pocket hematoma - Pneumothorax - Hemothorax - Myocardial perforation/cardiac tamponade - Massive pulmonary embolism - Arteriovenous (AV) fistula - Vascular laceration	- Phlebitis - Thrombophlebitis - Tricuspid regurgitation - Pacemaker malfunction (failure to pace, failure to sense, failed capture, dysrhythmia, lead fracture) - Pocket infection - Lead dislodgement	- Pacemaker malfunction - Tricuspid regurgitation - Endocarditis - Lead dislodgement - Pocket erosion - Twiddler syndrome - Myocardial perforation - Pectoral muscle stimulation - Intercostal/diaphragm pacing - Thrombosis (access vein, inferior vena cava, right atrium)

mechanical telescoping sheaths, powered sheaths, snares, locking stylets and laser/radiofrequency devices [5, 6]. However, regardless of the technique used, clinicians must be prepared to deal with the procedure which may vary from a relatively simple lead extraction to an extremely complicated one. Thus the procedure requires expert clinicians, with careful planning along with meticulous patient preparation, to prevent and manage complications that may arise during pacemaker lead extraction (Table 2) [5, 6].

The principle of patience is crucial when caring for patients with LC. Resolution of conduction abnormalities can take upwards of 10 days (range 3–42) with appropriate antibiotics [6]. Thus, allowing adequate time for the recovery of the conduction system, is vital to circumvent the disease and avoid unnecessary implantation of a permanent device. If a permanent pacemaker has been implanted as part of the management of LC, treating physicians should arrange explantation as soon as possible, as long as their conduction abnormality has resolved.

3   Review of Algorithm

The diagnosis of LC should ideally be made while the patient is still in the hospital. In some cases, patients are discharged before a formal diagnosis of LC is made, depending on the availability and speed of serological testing but also depending on whether the diagnosis of LC was considered. Patients diagnosed with LC should be started promptly on guideline-directed antibiotics. The Infectious Diseases Society of America (IDSA) recommends a 14–21 day course of antibiotics as covered in Chap. 8. Early treatment is associated with a good prognosis [1].

Following the treatment of LC with antibiotics, patients who have undergone placement of a permanent pacemaker device should receive early follow-up by an electrophysiologist and/or device clinic. The algorithm published by Wamboldt

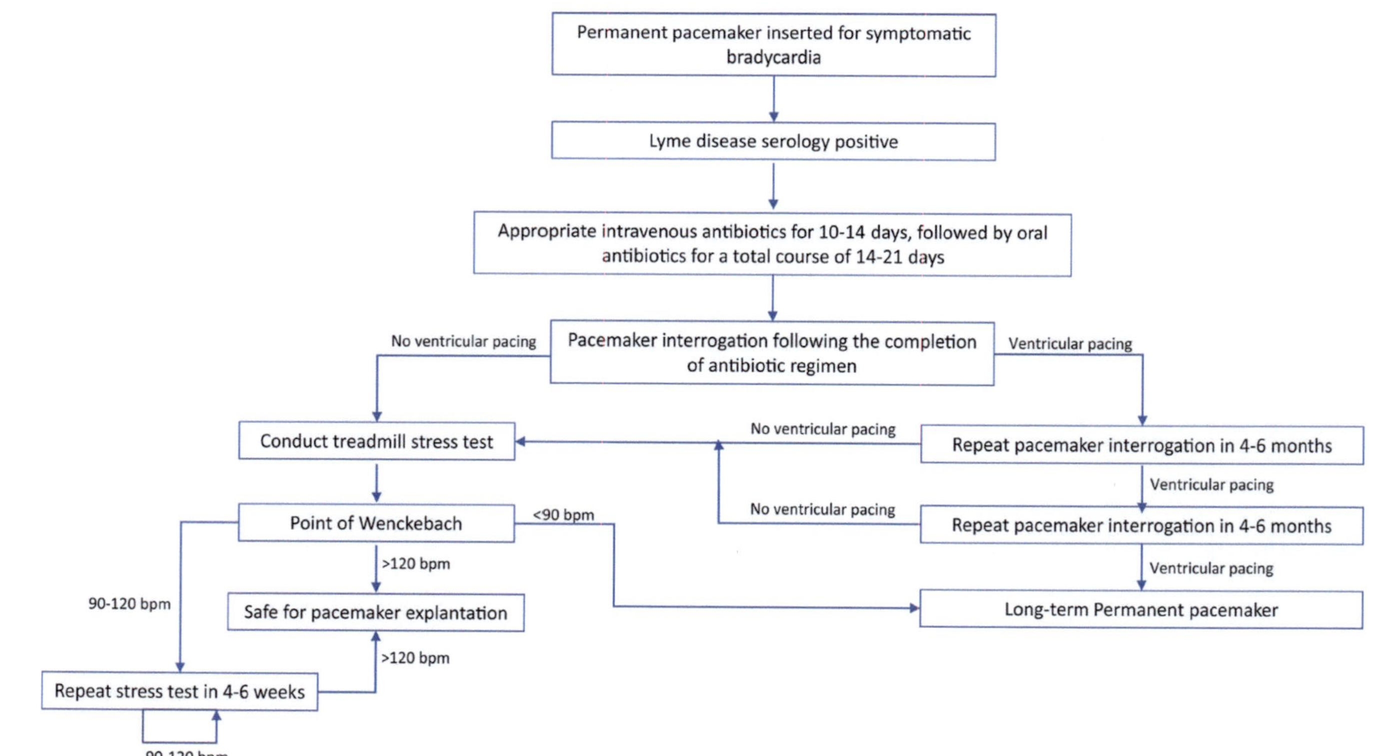

Fig. 1 Algorithm for permanent pacemaker explantation in Lyme carditis (JACC Case Reports)

Table 2 Complications associated with pacemaker extraction

Complications associated with pacemaker lead extraction
Pericardial effusion
Venous thrombosis
Migrated lead fragment
Hematoma/bleeding
AV fistula
Pulmonary embolism
Pneumothorax
Cardiac/respiratory arrest
Cerebrovascular accident
Vascular laceration
Death

et al. should be followed to facilitate the safe explantation of cardiac pacemakers for those where it is deemed clinically appropriate (Fig. 1) [2]. The first step is to organize a pacemaker interrogation, to assess for the presence of ventricular pacing. If ventricular pacing persists, a follow-up should be arranged in 4–6 months for re-interrogation. If the patient continues to be reliant on the pacemaker after two further assessments, they will likely require long-term pacing. Ongoing follow-up should be arranged by their cardiac device clinic and/or cardiologist.

For patients with no evidence of ventricular pacing on pacemaker interrogation, treadmill stress testing should be pursued to evaluate AV node function. A modified Bruce protocol should be used with continuous cardiac monitoring. If the patient can maintain 1:1 AV conduction at a heart rate greater than 120 beats per minute (bpm), device explantation can be safely arranged. If the patient is unable to maintain 1:1 AV conduction at a heart rate greater than 120 bpm, stress testing should be repeated. Those who are unable to achieve 1:1 conduction over a heart rate of 90bpm, will likely require a permanent pacemaker.

4   Conclusion

Pacemaker explantation is a safe option for patients who have undergone permanent pacemaker implantation as part of the management of LC. Explantation should ideally be performed within the first year. Patients should have received a full course of guideline-directed antibiotics, should have no evidence of ventricular pacing on device interrogation and should retain 1:1 AV conduction on treadmill stress testing.

References

1. Yeung C, Baranchuk A. Diagnosis and treatment of lyme carditis: JACC review topic of the week. J Am Coll Cardiol. 2019;73(6):717–26.
2. Wamboldt R, Wang C, Miller JC, Enriquez A, Yeung C, Chacki S, Foisy M, Baranchuk A. Pacemaker explantation in patients with lyme carditis. JACC Case Rep. 2022;4(10):613–6.
3. Lantos PM, Rumbaugh J, Bockenstedt LK, et al. Clinical practice guidelines by the infectious diseases society of America (IDSA), American academy of neurology (AAN), and American college of rheumatology (ACR): 2020 guidelines for the prevention, diagnosis and treatment of lyme disease. Clin Infect Dis. 2021;71:e1–48.
4. Bush LM, Vazquez-Pertejo MT. Tick borne illness-Lyme disease. Dis Mon. 2018;64:195–212.
5. Bongiorni MG, Burri H, Deharo JC, Starck C, Kennergren C, Saghy L, Rao A, Tascini C, Lever N, Kutarski A, Lozano IF, Strathmore N, Costa R, Epstein L, Love C, Blomstrom-Lundqvist C. EHRA expert consensus statement on lead extraction: recommendations on definitions, endpoints, research trial design, and data collection requirements for clinical scientific studies and registries: endorsed by APHRS/HRS/LAHRS. Eur Soc Cardiol. 2018;20:1217.
6. Perez AA, Woo FW, Tsang DC, Carrillo RG. Transvenous lead extractions: current approaches and future trends. Arrhythm Electrophysiol Rev. 2018;7(3):210–7.

Modelling Late Disseminated Lyme Carditis

Mehras Motamed, Kiera Liblik, Juan Maria Farina,
Alison W. Rebman, Cheryl B. Novak, John N. Aucott,
and Adrian Baranchuk

Abstract

The development of Lyme disease-dilated cardiomyopathy likely involves three pathophysiological processes, including direct spirochetal invasion, dysfunctional immune response, and autoimmune processes. The association between Lyme disease and dilated cardiomyopathy remains tentative due to heterogenous results of existing studies. Further high-quality investigations are required to elucidate this potential link. Antibiotic therapy in patients with suspected Lyme disease-dilated cardiomyopathy may significantly improve clinical status and cardiac function, but its benefits are likely limited in late stages of the disease process.

M. Motamed (✉)
Department of Medicine, University of Toronto, Toronto, ON, Canada
e-mail: mmotamed@qmed.ca

K. Liblik · A. Baranchuk
Division of Cardiology, Department of Medicine, Kingston Health Science Center, Queen's University, Kingston, ON, Canada
e-mail: 14kl3@queensu.ca

A. Baranchuk
e-mail: Adrian.Baranchuk@kingstonhsc.ca

J. M. Farina
Department of Cardiovascular and Thoracic Surgery, Mayo Clinic Arizona, Phoenix, AZ, USA

A. W. Rebman · C. B. Novak · J. N. Aucott
Lyme Disease Research Center, Division of Rheumatology, Department of Medicine, Johns Hopkins University School of Medicine, Baltimore, MD, USA
e-mail: arebman1@jhmi.edu

C. B. Novak
e-mail: cnovak7@jhmi.edu

J. N. Aucott
e-mail: jaucott2@jhmi.edu

Keywords

Lyme carditis • Lyme disease • Lyme cardiomyopathy • Dilated cardiomyopathy • Heart failure

1 Introduction

Lyme disease (LD) progresses in discrete phases which are classically labeled as (i) early localized LD, (ii) early disseminated LD, and (iii) late disseminated LD. Lyme carditis (LC) is a well described cardiovascular phenomenon in early disseminated LD which is characterized by high-degree atrioventricular block (up to 10% of LC cases). Rarely, myocarditis and pericarditis may occur. However, the chronic sequalae of LC and its potential long-term consequences in late disseminated LD are poorly understood.

Late disseminated LD occurs months to years after initial infection [1]. One possible manifestation of late disseminated LC is dilated cardiomyopathy (DCM). DCM is characterized by left ventricular or biventricular enlargement, dilation, and impaired contractile function. This potential link was first identified by Stanek et al. in 1990 who described a case of a 54-year-old man with DCM and *B. burgdorferi* isolated on endomyocardial biopsy (EMB) [2].

Emerging literature continues to associate LD with the development of subsequent DCM. Accordingly, several case reports and observational studies have sparked further interest in this research area. However, this association remains controversial [3]. The aim of this chapter is to review the available literature on cardiac manifestations in late disseminated LD with commentary on pathophysiological processes, a review of the current literature, and future directions for research.

2 Pathophysiology

2.1 Pathogenesis of Cardiac Damage in *Borrelia* Infection

The mechanisms by which LD leads to cardiac damage have not been fully elucidated. Several have been postulated, including direct invasion of cardiac tissue by *B. burgdorferi*, immune evasion, dysfunctional immune response, and autoimmune processes resulting in chronic inflammation. A summary of the hypothesized pathophysiology of LD-DCM is provided in Fig. 1 [3].

B. burgdorferi evades both the innate and adaptive immune system by regulating the expression of its surface proteins. Examples in the outer surface protein E-related proteins and complement regulator-acquiring surface proteins. These proteins bind and inhibit C3b, which allows the spirochete to inactivate the complement cascade and resist complement-mediated killing. Further evasion of the host adaptive immune system and IgM-mediated killing in the early phase of infection

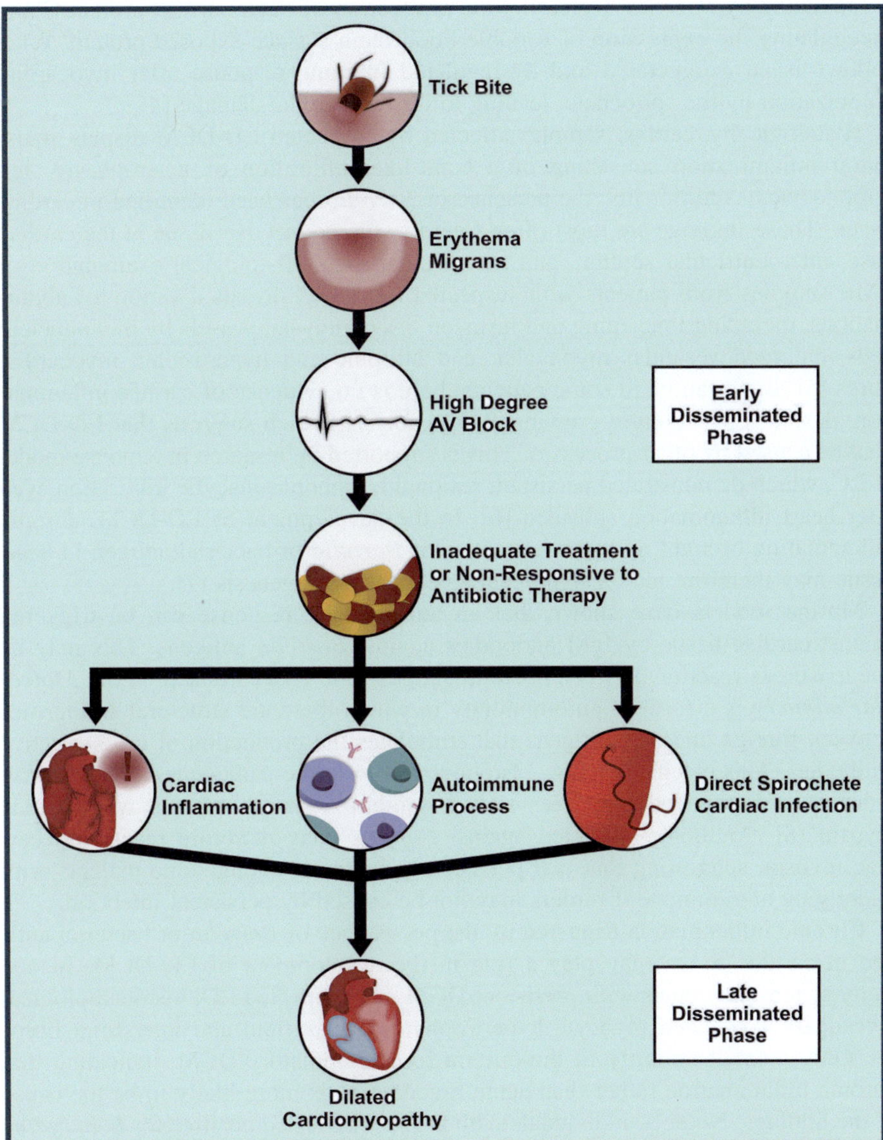

Fig. 1 Possible pathophysiological mechanisms involved in the development of LD-DCM. As a potential late manifestation of LD, LD-DCM may occur due to chronic inflammation, autoimmune processes, and direct spirochete infection of cardiac tissue

is facilitated by *Borrelia* decreasing the production of outer surface protein C and upregulating the expression of variable lipoprotein surface-exposed protein. What follows is an exaggerated and dysregulated immune response after myocardial colonization by the spirochete, leading to further cardiac damage [4].

Histologically, cardiac samples affected by suspected LD-DCM display transmural inflammation consisting of a band-like infiltration of macrophages and lymphocytes. Additionally, the presence of *Borrelia* has been identified in cardiac tissue. These findings are most often found in the connective tissue at the cardiac base, interventricular septum, and perivascular area. Histological examination of EMB samples from patients with suspected LD-DCM reveals a variety of abnormalities, including thickening and invasion of endomysial vessels by mononuclear cells, enlarged vesicular myonuclei, and atrophic and hypertrophic myocardial fibres [5]. Importantly, in some patients there is no evidence of cardiac inflammation, despite EMB culture growing *B. burgdorferi*, which suggests that LD-DCM may be caused by other processes. This is supported by research in a mouse model of LC, which demonstrated persistent residual lymphoplasmacytic infiltration even after heart inflammation subsided [6]. In the development of LD-DCM, chronic inflammation brought on by the presence of *Borrelia* or bacterial antigen in heart tissue may therefore play a significant role in its pathogenesis [7].

Murine models have shown that an autoimmune response can be triggered against cardiac tissue by IgM antibodies against *Borrelia* antigens. This may be due to a cross-reaction between *Borrelia* antigens and host cardiac proteins. ***Molecular mimicry*** is a form of autoimmunity in which there are structural similarities between foreign and self-antigens that stimulates the production of cross-reactive antibodies. This mechanism may also be involved in the pathogenesis of *Borrelia*-induced cardiomyopathy, as outer-surface protein A shares epitopes with cardiac myosin [8]. Antibodies directed against *Borrelia* may therefore react with cardiac myosin, suggesting that that persistent symptoms among some patients with underlying autoimmune disorders may not be caused by persistent infection.

Chronic inflammation triggered by the persistence of *Borrelia* or bacterial antigen in cardiac tissue may play a role in the development of LD-DCM. In one study of ten individuals with persistent DCM and suspected LD, histopathological investigation revealed myocyte hypertrophy, vacuolization, and interstitial fibrosis. Only a small minority fit the criteria for inflammatory DCM, indicating that chronic inflammation rather than acute myocarditis is more likely to be the cause of the findings. Notably, individuals with DCM who tested positive for *B. burgdorferi* had a greater incidence of autoimmune diseases. This is also consistent with research in murine models showing that autoimmune-susceptible animals had prolonged *B. burgdorferi* persistence in cardiac tissue. Although more research is needed to fully articulate the role of molecular mimicry in the development of LC, the presence of structural similarities between OspA and cardiac myosin is a hypothesis-generating finding [7].

Finally, it is important to consider patient risk factors and how they may mediate the risk of late cardiac manifestations of LD. These include pre-existing cardiac conditions, autoimmune conditions, and immunocompromise. Myocardial injury is often followed by tissue necrosis and scar tissue development, a process partly regulated by the extracellular protein decorin. Decorin is upregulated to facilitate the remodelling process. *Borrelia* spirochetes adhere to the extracellular matrix via decorin-binding protein A on the spirochete's outer membrane in the disseminated phase of Lyme infection. Both decorin and decorin-binding protein A are necessary for cardiac infection by *Borrelia*, as demonstrated by reduced tropism to cardiac tissue in decorin knock-out mice [7]. It is therefore likely that multiple pathways are involved in the development of LD-DCM.

2.2   Lyme Persistence—Lessons Learned and Applied to Late Lyme Carditis

It has been well-demonstrated in several animal models and human studies that B. *burgdorferi* can survive the initial host immune response [9]. Research on primates has demonstrated that morphologically intact and metabolically active spirochetes in the brain and heart may endure antibiotic therapy. Patients who exhibit symptoms after appropriate therapy have raised suspicion that spirochetes may survive following treatment in humans. However, it remains unclear whether human patients who experience LD symptoms after antibiotic treatment still have an active infection. This is complicated by the lack of accurate diagnostic methods to detect whether infection has been eliminated in LD patients. Thus, it remains unknown to what extent ongoing infection, poor clearance of borrelial antigens, and/or autoimmune reactivity contribute to ongoing LD symptoms, including late cardiac manifestations.

It was initially thought that *B. burgdorferi* spirochetes isolated in patients treated appropriately with antibiotics were non-viable and therefore infection could not be persistent. This was based primarily on the fact that in LD, only *B. burgdorferi* genetic material, antigen, or non-culturable spirochetes have been detected following antibiotic treatment, with rare exception. However, evidence now exists that antibiotic-treated *B. burgdorferi* spirochetes can be persistent and, importantly, metabolically active [9]. *Borrelia* can alter its morphology to atypical dormant spirochete forms known as ***persisters*** in response to hostile environmental conditions [9]. Persisters can survive aggressive antibiotic therapy and transform into motile forms in favourable environments. Despite being non-culturable following antibiotic therapy, these persistent spirochetes retain the ability to alter the expression of bacterial genes in the infected host. These large-scale changes in gene expression include increased expression of pro-inflammatory cytokines and chemokines, as demonstrated in spirochetes localized to the dura mater of the brain. Persistent cystic forms of *B. burgdorferi* have been isolated from the cerebral cortex of patients with chronic Lyme neuroborreliosis, which may explain cases of persisting infection. One investigation on 33 patients with DCM identified spirochetes 10 patients on EMB analysis. Importantly, some of these spirochetes were identified in pleomorphic and atypical cystic forms, suggesting that persistent

Lyme infection of cardiac tissue may be involved in the pathogenesis of LD-DCM [10].

3   Overview of Evidence

3.1   Lyme and Dilated Cardiomyopathy—An Overview of the Literature

Eleven observational studies have been conducted thus far to try and explain the association between LD and DCM with heterogeneous results. All participants had pre-existing DCM. In line with the epidemiology of Lyme infection, the participants in these observational studies were usually more male than female, with mean ages ranging from 42 to 58 years. A recent systematic review has examined this relationship in detail [3].

All investigations implicating LD as a possible cause of DCM have been conducted among central European populations in endemic regions. Early reports relied primarily on seropositivity to make this association. In an Austrian study on patients with chronic idiopathic DCM, 19 of 72 were shown to be seropositive for IgG antibodies against *B. burgdorferi* compared to only seven patients of 55 with DCM due to coronary artery disease and five of 55 healthy control patients [11]. Several subsequent investigations from the same group found similar results, with one study finding 26% of patients (n = 46) with known idiopathic DCM being IgG seropositive against B. *burgdorferi* [12] and another finding nearly identical levels (24%) [13]. At least one of these patients had what appeared to be spirochete-like forms isolated from cardiac tissue. More recently, four observational studies utilized polymerase chain reaction (PCR) of EMB samples or peripheral PCR utilizing blood samples, as well as electron microscopy, to supplement serology findings. These investigations identified a significant prevalence of *B. burgdorferi* sensu lato genome in patients with suspected LD-DCM [5, 14–16]. In fact, one study detected *B. burgdorferi* sensu lato DNA in the EMB samples in all participants with DCM (n = 17). [14]

Studies conducted in the United States and United Kingdom have cast doubt on the association between LD and DCM. Four investigations, from both Europe and North America, have failed to show a connection between Lyme borreliosis and DCM. A study in an endemic region of the United States on 175 patients with DCM showed no significant difference in the seropositivity between patients with idiopathic DCM and ischemic DCM [17]. Similarly, in a study in the United Kingdom, although 8.2% of patients with DCM were seropositive against *B. burgdorferi*, this was not significantly greater than in the control groups. Additionally, immunoblot analysis was negative on all samples with positive enzyme-linked immunosorbent assay (ELISA) [18]. In one study in an endemic region of Germany, 12.5% of sera samples in patients with end-stage DCM were IgG-positive, which is not significantly higher than expected for populations in endemic regions for LD. Importantly, the *B. burgdorferi* OpsA gene was undetected in any patient with DCM using a nested PCR technique [19]. More recently, a second German investigation examined the frequency of *B. burgdorferi*, *B. afzelii*, or *B. garinii* DNA in EMB samples from 64 patients with suspected inflammatory DCM who had positive *B. burgdorferi* IgM serology. PCR was used to identify *Borrelia* DNA in EMB samples, but found no evidence of the genomes of *B. burgdorferi*, *B. afzelii*, or *B. garinii* [20].

It is possible that *B. burgdorferi* only manifests in early stages of DCM and disappears from the myocardium over time. Further, in the absence of the active infectious agent, persistent post-inflammatory reactions generated by spirochetes may be the source of the cardiac structural and functional abnormalities seen in end-stage DCM. As all studies that did find a connection between LD and DCM were conducted in endemic areas of Europe, where B. *afzelii* and B. *garinii* are the common pathogens responsible for human LD, this discrepancy between the studies may also be explained by the geographical distribution of LD. *B. garinii* and *B. burgdorferi* appear to be more neurotropic and confers a stronger risk of neurological disease than *B. afezlii*. Infections with these strains are associated with different inflammatory profiles. For example, *B. burgdorferi* strains found in North America are associated with a T helper cell-1 adaptive immune response and elicit a higher level of cytokines and chemokines than their strains found in Europe [21]. It is unclear if these European strains produce a more indolent, subclinical infection that over a prolonged period could lead to the development of DCM. Additionally, *B burgdorferi* is not uniformly distributed in cardiac tissue. In murine models infected with *B. burgdorferi,* the spirochetes localized primarily to the cardiac apex. Therefore, samples might have been taken from regions devoid of B. *burgdorferi*. However, this remains speculative and the association between LD and DCM remains elusive.

3.2   Lyme Disease-Dilated Cardiomyopathy and Antibiotics

Perhaps the strongest evidence in support of an association between LD and the development of DCM is the improvement in cardiac function or the complete reversal of DCM with the administration of antibiotics. The majority of investigations to date have found that antibiotic treatment with or without conventional heart failure drugs significantly enhance cardiac function, reverses pathological cardiac remodelling, and improves clinical status [13, 15, 16, 20]. Conversely, two studies have found no improvement in left ventricular function or pathological remodeling after a standard course of ceftriaxone in patients with LD-DCM [5, 17].

How can we make sense of these contradictory findings? One hypothesis is that early antibiotic therapy in suspected LD-DCM could reduce inflammation prior to the development of permanent cardiac damage associated with chronic DCM. This is supported by a study that found a moderate correlation between the length of cardiac symptoms and improvement in cardiac function with antibiotics in eleven patients with *B. burgdorferi*-positive DCM. Patients with shorter DCM symptoms duration showed greater improvements in cardiac function [13]. It is therefore possible that antibiotics in suspected LD-DCM may provide clinical benefits to patients only up until a certain point in the disease course.

3.3 Diagnostic Issues and Considerations

It is crucial to consider the difficulty of diagnosing LD in patients with idiopathic DCM when assessing the validity of the findings in studies investigating the link between LD and DCM. The existing literature on suspected LD-DCM has utilized several techniques to diagnose *Borrelia* infection. These includes ELISA alone, standard two-tier testing (STTT) (which combines ELISA with confirmatory immunoblotting), PCR (of blood and an EMB sample), and electron microscopy. Due to the low sensitivity of ELISA in the early stages of widespread LD and the post-treatment convalescent period, serological testing has been ineffective in establishing a causal relationship between LD and DCM. Additionally, it can be difficult to determine whether seropositivity is due to past or recent/current infection as both IgM and IgG *B. burgdorferi*-specific antibody response can last for years after the initial infection has been cleared. Other widely acknowledged limitations of serological testing include that these tests can cross-react with non-*B. burgdorferi* antibodies and their susceptibility to variable results depending on the choice of antigens used in the first-tier test, and their requirement for interpretation, particularly regarding the Western immunoblot assay, which may introduce bias. Therefore, the conclusions that can be drawn from the existing literature is limited and must be taken cautiously [3].

Although STTT is still the preferred diagnostic test, the absence of a standardized diagnostic methodology in the literature adds another layer of complexity when evaluating the relationship between LD and DCM. Recent investigations have employed the more sensitive approach of PCR testing and discovered a considerably greater incidence of *B. burgdorferi* in patients with DCM [5, 14–16, 19, 20]. This is due to the variable predictive value of ELISA serum assay and confirmatory immunoblotting. The *B. burgdorferi* genome was found in the myocardium of patients with presumably new onset DCM utilizing quantitative and qualitative PCR analysis and electron microscopy for direct spirochete detection. When compared to controls, the myocardium of DCM patients had a considerably higher rate of *B. burgdorferi* genome, according to quantitative PCR analysis of EMB samples [5].

One study found that a combination of western blot and qualitative serum PCR is the test with the greatest positive predictive value for *B. burgdorferi* sensu lato in EMB. Quantitative PCR was the gold standard for confirming *B. burgdorferi* in the endocardium, whereas a positive ELISA had just 50% sensitivity. *B. Burgdorferi* may become more closely associated to the development of DCM with the application of serum PCR and western blot [16]. However, due to the subpar assessment of PCR testing and electron microscopy in identifying *Borrelia* infection, these results should be regarded with care. As such, the International Diseases Society of America does not routinely recommend PCR testing of blood samples in

Table 1 Diagnostic methods utilized in investigations on suspected LD-DCM

Diagnostic method	Description	Advantages	Disadvantages
Standard two-tiered test	Consists of ELISA, which detects the presence of both IgM and IgG antibodies to *borrelia* Positive results are confirmed with immunoblotting	Cost-effective Readily available in most testing centers	Variable and generally poor sensitivity Difficult to determine whether seropositivity is due to recent/current or pre or recent/current infection
Polymerase chain reaction	Detects *borrelia* DNA in peripheral tissue (blood) or cardiac tissue	Cost-effective PCR can be used on a variety of testable tissue (e.g., blood, cerebrospinal fluid, cardiac tissue) The application of multiple PCR assays to the same sample can improve sensitivity	PCR for *B. burgdorferi* is not standardized. sensitivity varies according to the specific technique used The use of *B. burgdorferi* PCR directly on blood samples is substantially less sensitive compared with PCR performed on skin lesion samples in early infection Typically available only at large reference laboratories
Light microscopy	Quantitative method of detecting *borrelia* in cardiac tissue through use of microscopy	Allows for the direct detection of *borrelia*	Direct identification of spirochetes in tissue slides is limited due to low *borrelia* load Requires endomyocardial biopsy, which is invasive and rarely performed in clinical practice Heterogenous distribution of *borrelia* in cardiac tissue reduces sensitivity

patients with suspected LD. Diagnostic methods employed in suspected LD-DCM including their advantages and disadvantages are summarized in Table 1.

4   Future Directions and Conclusions

Several observational studies support the association between LD and DCM. Though, this relationship is not supported by randomized trials or definitive evidence of a pathophysiological relationship. Additionally, high quality studies are required to determine the most appropriate choice, route, and duration of antibiotic therapy in patients with suspected LD-DCM. Due to a lack of long-term follow-up research on LC patients or the possibility of patients receiving subpar LD treatment, the true prevalence of DCM in late disseminated LD may be underreported.

To assess if *B. burgdorferi* is a causal agent of DCM, whether antibiotic therapy would improve associated clinical outcomes, it is critical to perform large-scale longitudinal investigations and randomized controlled trials3].

Our understanding of the pathophysiology of LD-DCM remains poor and the relative importance of direct spirochetal infection, immune dysfunction, and autoimmune processes remains unclear. Preclinical investigations in murine models can help to better characterize how *Borrelia* invades cardiac tissue, promotes inflammation, and evades the immune system. Recently, the use of bioluminescent *Borrelia* has been employed to directly analyze the spatiotemporal expression and regulation of *Borrelia* genes, allowing for real-time evaluation of *Borrelia* load during murine infection. Analysis of the kinetics of infection of the different *Borrelia* genospecies and alterations in gene expression of *Borrelia* in cardiac tissue could be highly beneficial to our understanding of the pathophysiology of LD-DCM.

At present, clinicians may therefore rely on EMB, but this remains an invasive and potentially dangerous procedure that is not routinely used. Therefore, more investigations are required to identify biomarkers and unique features of LD-DCM to improve diagnostic accuracy and clinical management.

References

1. Yeung C, Mendoza I, Echeverria LE, Baranchuk A. Chagas' cardiomyopathy and Lyme carditis: lessons learned from two infectious diseases affecting the heart. Trends Cardiovasc Med. 2021;31:233–9.
2. Stanek G, Klein J, Bittner R, Glogar D. Isolation of Borrelia burgdorferi from the myocardium of a patient with longstanding cardiomyopathy. N Engl J Med. 1990;322:249–52.
3. Motamed M, Liblik K, Miranda-Arboleda AF, et al. Disseminated Lyme disease and dilated cardiomyopathy: a systematic review. Trends Cardiovasc Med. 2022;S1050–1738(22):00077–9.
4. Anderson C, Brissette CA. The Brilliance of Borrelia: mechanisms of host immune evasion by lyme disease-causing spirochetes. Pathogens (Basel, Switzerland) 2021;10.
5. Kubánek M, Šramko M, Berenová D, et al. Detection of Borrelia burgdorferi sensu lato in endomyocardial biopsy specimens in individuals with recent-onset dilated cardiomyopathy. Eur J Heart Fail. 2012;14:588–96.
6. Armstrong AL, Barthold SW, Persing DH, Beck DS. Carditis in Lyme disease susceptible and resistant strains of laboratory mice infected with Borrelia burgdorferi. Am J Tropical Med Hygiene. 1992;47:249–58.
7. Hyde JA. Borrelia burgdorferi keeps moving and carries on: a review of borrelial dissemination and invasion. Front Immunol. 2017;8:114.
8. Raveche ES, Schutzer SE, Fernandes H, et al. Evidence of Borrelia autoimmunity-induced component of Lyme carditis and arthritis. J Clin Microbiol. 2005;43:850–6.
9. Rudenko N, Golovchenko M, Kybicova K, Vancova M. Metamorphoses of Lyme disease spirochetes: phenomenon of Borrelia persisters. Parasit Vectors. 2019;12:237.
10. Bartůnek P, Gorican K, Mrázek V, et al. Lyme borreliosis infection as a cause of dilated cardiomyopathy. Prague Med Rep. 2006;107:213–26.
11. Stanek G, Klein J, Bittner R, Glogar D. Borrelia burgdorferi as an etiologic agent in chronic heart failure? Scand J Infect Dis Suppl. 1991;77:85–7.

12. Klein J, Stanek G, Bittner R, Horvat R, Holzinger C, Glogar D. Lyme borreliosis as a cause of myocarditis and heart muscle disease. Eur Heart J. 1991;12 Suppl D:73–5.
13. Gasser R, Fruhwald F, Schumacher M, et al. Reversal of Borrelia burgdorferi associated dilated cardiomyopathy by antibiotic treatment? Cardiovasc Drugs Ther. 1996;10:351–60.
14. Bartůněk P, Gorican K, Veiser T, Táborský M, Hulínská D. Significance of Borrelia infection in development of dilated cardiomypathy (a pilot study). Prague Med Rep. 2007;108:339–47.
15. Kuchynka P, Palecek T, Havranek S, et al. Recent-onset dilated cardiomyopathy associated with Borrelia burgdorferi infection. Herz. 2015;40:892–7.
16. Palecek T, Kuchynka P, Hulinska D, et al. Presence of Borrelia burgdorferi in endomyocardial biopsies in patients with new-onset unexplained dilated cardiomyopathy. Med Microbiol Immunol. 2010;199:139–43.
17. Sonnesyn SW, Diehl SC, Johnson RC, Kubo SH, Goodman JL. A prospective study of the seroprevalence of Borrelia burgdorferi infection in patients with severe heart failure. Am J Cardiol. 1995;76:97–100.
18. Rees DH, Keeling PJ, McKenna WJ, Axford JS. No evidence to implicate Borrelia burgdorferi in the pathogenesis of dilated cardiomyopathy in the United Kingdom. Br Heart J. 1994;71:459–61.
19. Suedkamp M, Lissel C, Eiffert H, et al. Cardiac myocytes of hearts from patients with end-stage dilated cardiomyopathy do not contain Borrelia Burgdorferi DNA. Am Heart J. 1999;138:269–72.
20. Karatolios K, Maisch B, Pankuweit S. Suspected inflammatory cardiomyopathy. Prevalence of Borrelia burgdorferi in endomyocardial biopsies with positive serological evidence. Herz. 2015;40 Suppl 1:91–5.
21. Cerar T, Strle F, Stupica D, et al. Differences in genotype, clinical features, and inflammatory potential of borrelia burgdorferi sensu stricto strains from Europe and the United States. Emerg Infect Dis. 2016;22:818–27.

Into the Future: Strategies for the Next 5–10 Years

Adrian Baranchuk, Rachel Wamboldt, and Chang Nancy Wang

Abstract

Research on Lyme disease and Lyme carditis is rapidly evolving, with new evidence constantly emerging on the diagnosis and treatment of LC. Future areas of research include prevention of Lyme complications, potential vaccine development for Lyme disease, and studies on the long-term effects of Lyme carditis. Interprofessional collaboration and patient participation is key in advancing future knowledge on Lyme disease.

Keywords

Lyme disease • Lyme carditis • Interprofessional collaboration

Several aspects pertaining to our knowledge about Lyme disease (LD) and specifically Lyme carditis (LC) are rapidly evolving. These areas include a better understanding of pathophysiological mechanisms that would allow the development of new therapeutic targets [1].

The complexity of this infectious disease includes multiple factors: from the scientific and medical-related aspects of the disease to the social and political determinants [2]. Several years ago, LD entered this complex arena and has slowly but firmly evolved to include many invested parties into it's research, treatment and

A. Baranchuk (✉) · R. Wamboldt · C. N. Wang
Division of Cardiology, Kingston Health Science Center, Queen's University, Kingston, ON, Canada
e-mail: Adrian.Baranchuk@kingstonhsc.ca

R. Wamboldt
e-mail: 17reaw@queensu.ca

C. N. Wang
e-mail: chwang@qmed.ca

prevention. It was the medical community that first recognized the importance of further research on this topic. This was soon followed by the incredible work of multiple non-governmental organizations (NGOs) as well as patients and families, fighting for their rights and supporting new initiatives to improve the quality of life for those chronically affected by this condition; recognizing not only the value of prevention, but also the long-term consequences of this disease. As the chronic consequences of LD are not fully understood or accepted as definitive conditions, the impact on reduced work capacity, applications to disability programs and possible treatment options for the chronic symptoms LD, are still in the development phase [3]. This creates a lot of uncertainties for the patients suffering long-term LD and their families.

Several areas concerning the future of LD and LC are worth mentioning:

1. For LD prevention, the development of a proven and effective vaccine should be available for people living in endemic regions with frequent outdoors activity (professional or recreational). Efforts in this direction will reduce the annual burden of this disease. At the same time, permanent campaigns using all possible communication pathways (including active Social Media presence), advising on how to enjoy outdoor activities in a safe manner, should be prioritized by government authorities.
2. For LC prevention, rapid and full evaluation of EVERY case of suspected or confirmed LD should be mandatory. This should include a full cardiovascular exam, and a 12-lead surface ECG. The traditional prevalence of LC of 4–10% could be much higher if you obtain regular ECGs in all LD cases. Some of the initial ECG manifestations can be totally asymptomatic [4, 5].
3. For LC diagnosis and treatment, the implementation of the previously published algorithm is essential to treat this potentially reversible heart condition [1, 4]. For that purpose, the SILC score (see Chap. 7) should be widely promoted and be a mandatory component of medical/nursing/health science education at early stages of a trainee's careers [6]. Currently, the CDC (Centers for Disease Control and Prevention) website supports the use of this algorithm, which is the only one in existence for the diagnosis and treatment of LC [7], however, failure to detect it continues to be a world-wide clinical problem. Educational platforms teaching how to suspect and deal with LC are paramount to reduce the number of underdiagnosed patients and the potential catastrophic consequences [8].
4. For LC progression into a chronic condition, there is ongoing research to better understand how unrecognized or poorly treated early disseminated LC could evolve into a chronic cardiomyopathy [3]. Research models are being developed to prove this concept, and to design medical strategies to avoid these long-term consequences. In this regard, the identification of inflammatory markers or evidence of auto-immune aggression against specific heart structures (i.e. conduction system), are essential to advance innovative medical options (see Chap. 18). The next years will be crucial to find potential new targets for treatment.

In summary, a new horizon is upon us in regards to LC research, that will continue to address the multiple challenges of this condition. Working in synchrony and respecting views from everybody involved, including the scientific and medical community, NGOs, patients and family advocates, will help us improve the quality of life of our communities. This entire book is dedicated to the thousands of individuals affected by this condition, with the hope of a better future in the next 5–10 years.

References

1. Yeung C, Baranchuk A. Diagnosis and treatment of Lyme carditis. J Am Coll Cardiol. 2019;73(6):717–26.
2. Gazendam N, Yeung C, Farina JM, Saldarriaga C, Mendoza I, Baranchuk A. Lyme and heart. In: Saldarriaga C, Baranchuk A, editors. The NET-heart book. London, UK: Elsevier; 2021. Chapter 8, p. 61–71.
3. Motamed M, Liblik K, Miranda-Arboleda AF, Wambolt R, Wang CN, Cingolani O, Rebman AW, Novak CB, Aucott JN, Farina JM, Baranchuk A. Disseminated Lyme disease and dilated cardiomyopathy: a systematic review. Trends Cardiovasc Med. 2022;S1050–1738(22)00077-9 (Epub ahead of print).
4. Yeung C, Baranchuk A. Systematic approach to the diagnosis and treatment of Lyme carditis and high-degree atrioventricular block. Healthcare (Basel). 2018;6(4)pii:E119.
5. Beach CM, Hart SA, Nowalk A, Feingold B, Kurland K, Arora G. Increasing burden of Lyme carditis in United States children's hospitals. Pediatr Cardiol. 2020;41(2):258–64.
6. Besant G, Wan D, Yeung C, Blakely C, Branscombe P, Suarez-Fuster L, Redfearn D, Simpson C, Abdollah H, Glover B, Baranchuk A. Suspicious index in Lyme carditis (SILC): systematic review and proposed new risk score. Clin Cardiol. 2018;41(12):1611–6.
7. https://www.cdc.gov/lyme/treatment/lymecarditis.html. Accessed 2023 Jan 6.
8. Saldarriaga C, Baranchuk A. The NET-heart book. London, UK: Elsevier; 2021.

Into the Future: Determining the True Prevalence of Lyme Carditis

Rachel Wamboldt and Adrian Baranchuk

Abstract

Standard reporting definitions of Lyme carditis do not adequately define the true prevalence of Lyme carditis. Asymptomatic patients with Lyme carditis require increased monitoring and follow-up to ensure resolution of cardiac inflammation. Future epidemiological research should include asymptomatic cases of Lyme carditis to determine the true prevalence of disease in adults.

Keywords

Lyme disease · Lyme carditis · Incidence · Follow-up · Monitoring · Prevalence

1   Introduction

Lyme carditis (LC) is thought to be a rare manifestation of Lyme disease. The conduction abnormalities associated with LC were first described by Dr. Allen Steere and colleagues in a retrospective case series of 20 patients in 1980 [1–3]. When the Centres for Disease Control and Prevention (CDC) defined LC in the mid-1980s, they included the descriptor of cardiac symptoms in their reporting definition [1, 4]. The prevalence at that time was reported to be around 10%; however, many of the reported cases were for palpitations alone, which represented 69% of cases [1, 4]. This definition was thought to be too broad and over-estimated the true prevalence of LC.

R. Wamboldt (✉) · A. Baranchuk
76 Stuart Street, Kingston, Ontario K7L 3N6, Canada
e-mail: 17reaw@queensu.ca

A. Baranchuk
e-mail: Adrian.Baranchuk@kingstonhsc.ca

Lyme disease (LD) became a reportable disease in the United States in 1991 [5]. That same year, the CDC introduced a standard reporting definition for LC of acute high-grade (2nd-degree or 3rd-degree) atrioventricular(AV) conduction defect and sometimes myocarditis, that resolves in days to weeks [6]. This definition remains today [7]. Despite standardized reporting for LD cases in the United States, the reporting of cardiac manifestations has been suboptional [1]. Between 2001 and 2010, a total of 256,373 cases of Lyme disease were reported to the CDC; of these, only 68% included clinical information [8]. Only 1.1% were identified as cases of LC [8].

It is evident that the historical definitions of LC need to be updated in keeping with the current information available on the clinical manifestation of the disease. It is not enough to capture only those with 2nd and 3rd degree AV blocks. We need to be aware of patients presenting with silent disease to prevent the morbidity, and rarely, the mortality that can result if LC is allowed to progress without appropriate monitoring and treatment.

2   Discussion

The estimated incidence of LC in untreated adults is 0.3–4% in Europe and 1–10% in the United States [9–11]. The observed difference in LC between North American and Europe has been explained by Europe having less cardiotropic genospecies of *Borrelia burgdorferi s.1.*, such as *B. garinii* and *B.afzelii,* in comparison to the predominant *B. burgdorferi* in the United States. [12] These estimates are likely a gross under-representation of the true prevalence given the inconsistencies of reporting cardiac involvement in patients diagnosed with LD and the lack of systematic approach to rule out cardiac involvement as part of early disseminated LD. Asymptomatic patients, who may have first-degree AV block, bundle branch blocks and/or fascicular blocks, or mild cardiac inflammation, are not included in the reported cases to the CDC. In the pediatric population, ECG changes have been found in LD patients without cardiac symptoms [13, 14]. Patients with early disseminated disease are more likely to have ECG abnormalities than those presenting with early localized disease (e.g., erythema migrans alone) [13, 15–17]. A prospective study in asymptomatic pediatric patients with definite LD, showed that 29% (4/14) had ECG abnormalities [13]. This study suggested that even in asymptomatic patients, evaluation with ECG is useful to screen for cardiac manifestations of LD but also that we are missing the mark when it comes to estimating the true prevalence of LC.

Since the introduction of the definition for LC by the CDC in the 1990s, our understanding of this condition has evolved to include a greater spectrum of electrophysiological manifestations including sinus blocks, atrial fibrillation/flutter, fascicular blocks, atrioventricular delays (1st, 2nd and 3rd degree blocks), ST-T wave abnormalities, QT prolongation as well as ventricular arrhythmia [6, 16, 18–20]. We now understand that LC can also involve the myocardium, endocardium and pericardium to varying degrees [6, 16]. In addition, *B. burgorferi*

Table 1 Recommended definition for epidemiological studies about Lyme carditis

In a patient with confirmed (via serological testing) or highly suspicious presentation (based on exposure history or physical findings) for Lyme disease, Lyme carditis is defined as
(i) New conduction or rhythm abnormalities on 12-lead ECG **AND/OR**
(ii) Acute elevation in cardiac biomarkers, after exclusion of other possible causes **AND/OR**
(iii) Echocardiographic evidence of new dilated cardiomyopathy or valvulopathy

has also been isolated from the myocardium of patients with unexplained dilated cardiomyopathy (see Chap. 14 for *further details)* [17, 21, 22].

Our standard definition needs to be adjusted to be more inclusive of the current data on the clinical manifestations of LC. We propose that this definition includes clinical history, examination, and investigative data (Table 1) with emphasis on obtaining 12-lead ECG in all cases of confirmed or highly suspected LD. We also propose the inclusion of serological and cardiac biomarkers to further the delineate the true prevalence of disease, and to capture potential cases of myocarditis.

The cardiac manifestations of LD can progress rapidly and can be potentially fatal if allowed to progress untreated [16]. Identification of those individuals with conduction abnormalities is critical to help facilitate admission to hospital, cardiac monitoring, and treatment with intravenous antibiotics. We acknowledge that this algorithm requires validation; however given our current knowledge surrounding the progression of LC, this is the safest approach for patients (Fig. 1). We are currently finalizing a proposal to evaluate the true prevalence of LC in those presenting to the emergency department with confirmed or highly suspected LD. This study will also look to identify those with asymptomatic disease (i.e., no cardiovascular manifestations) to truly understand the prevalence of LC amongst adults infected with *B. burgdorferi*. We will be using the algorithm outlined in Fig. 1 to more accurately manage patients within our study. We suspect that the incidence of LC is higher than that estimated by historical definitions.

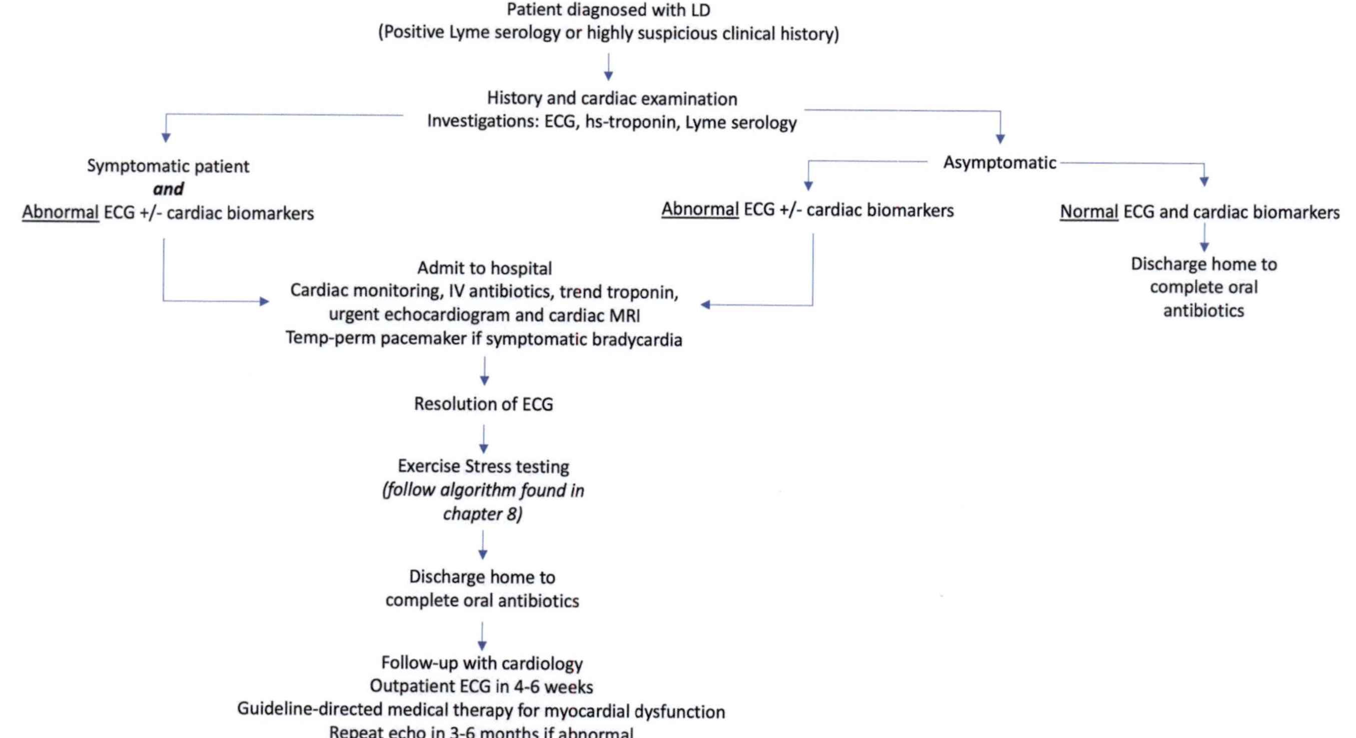

Fig. 1 Suggested management algorithm for patients diagnosed with Lyme disease and suspected Lyme carditis in the emergency department

3   Conclusion

A new investigative strategy is required to capture the true prevalence of LC. We need to transition away from historical definitions of the disease to incorporate our current knowledge on the diversity of clinical manifestations.

References

1. Robinson ML, Kobayashi T, Higgins Y, Calkins H, Melia MT. Lyme carditis. Inf Dis Clin North Am. 2015;29:255–68.
2. Steere AC, Batsford WP, Weinberg M, et al. Lyme carditis: cardiac abnormalities of Lyme disease. Ann Intern Med. 1980;93(1):8–16.
3. Fish AE, Pride YB, Pinto DS. Lyme carditis. Infect Dis Clin N Am. 2008;22:275–88.
4. Ciesielski CA, Markowitz LE, Horsley R, et al. Lyme disease surveillance in the united states, 1983–1986. Rev Infect Dis. 1989;11(Suppl 6):S1435–41.
5. Bush LM, Vazquez-Pertejo MT. Tick born illness- Lyme disease. Dis Mon. 2018;64(5):195–212.
6. Cox J, Krajden M. Cardiovascular manifestations of Lyme disease. Am Heart J. 1991;122:1449–55.
7. Centers for Disease Control and Prevention. Lyme Disease (Borrelia burgdorferi). National Notifiable Disease Surveillance System (NNDSS) [internet]. 2021. Available from: https://ndc. services.cdc.gov/case-definitions/lyme-disease-2022/.
8. Forrester JD, Meiman J, Mullins J, Nelson R, Ertel SH, Cartter M, Brown CM, Lijewski V, Schiffman E, Neitzel D, et al. Notes from the field: update on Lyme carditis, groups at high risk, and frequency of associated sudden cardiac death—United States. MMWR Morb Mortal Wkly Rep. 2014;63:982–3.
9. Radesich C, Del Mestre E, Medo K, Vitrella G, Manca P, Chiatto M, Castrichini M, Sinagra G. Lyme carditis: from pathophysiology to clinical management. Pathogens. 2022;11(582).
10. Steere AC, Strle F, Wormser GP, Hu LT, Branda JA, Hovius JWR, Li X, Mead PS. Lyme borreliosis. Nat Rev. 2016;2:1–18.
11. Centers for Disease Control and Prevention. Lyme carditis [internet]. 2022. Available from: https://www.cdc.gov/lyme/treatment/lymecarditis.html
12. O'Connell S, Granström M, Gray JS, Stanek G. Epidemiology of European Lyme borreliosis. Zentralblatt für Bakteriologie. 1998;287:229–40.
13. Welsh EJ, Cohn KA, Nigrovic LE, et al. Electrocardiograph abnormalities in children with Lyme meningitis. J Pediatric Infect Dis Soc. 2012;1:293–8.
14. Neville DN, Alexander ME, Bennett JE, Balamuth F, Garro A, Levas MN, Thompson AD, Kharbanda AB, Lewander DP, Dart AH, Nigrovic LE. Electrocardiogram as a Lyme disease screening test. J Pediatr. 2021;238–232.
15. Rubin DA, Sorbera C, Nikitin P, McAllister A, Wormser GP, Nadelman RB. Prospective evaluation of heart block complicating early Lyme disease. Pacing Clin Electrophysiol. 1992;15:252–5.
16. Costello JM, Alexander ME, Greco KM, Perez-Atayde AR, Laussen PC. Lyme carditis in children: presentation, predictive factors, and clinical course. Pediatrics. 2009;123:e835–41.
17. Mravljak M, Velnar T, Bricelj V, Ruzic-Sabljic E, Arnez M. Electrocardiographic findings in children with erythema migrans. Wien Klin Wochenschr. 2006;118:691–5.
18. Wan D, Blakely C, Branscombe P, Suarez-Fuster L, Glover B, Baranchuk A. Lyme carditis and high-degree atrioventricular block. Am J Cardiol. 2018;121(9):1102–4.
19. Gazendam N, Yeung C, Baranchuk A. Lyme carditis presenting as sick sinus syndrome. J Electrocardiol. 2020;59:65–7.

20. Maxwell N, Dryer MM, Baranchuk A, Vinocur JM. Phase 4 block of the right bundle branch suggesting His-Purkinje system involvement of Lyme carditis. Heart Rhythm Case Rep. 2020;7(2):112–6.
21. Motamed M, Liblik K, Miranda-Arboleda AF, Wambold R, Wang CN, Cingolani O, Rebman AW, Novak CB, Aucott JN, Farina JM, Baranchuk A. Disseminated Lyme disease and dilated cardiomyopathy: a systematic review. Trends Cardiovascular Med 2022; [in press] https://doi.org/10.1016/j.tcm.2022.05.010.
22. Stanek G, Klein J, Bittner R, Glogar D. Isolation of Borrelia burgdorferi from the myocardium of a patient with long- standing cardiomyopathy. N Engl J Med. 1990;322:249–52.

Into the Future: Research Prospects for Late Disseminated Lyme Carditis

Rachel Wamboldt, John Aucott, Oscar Cingolani, and Adrian Baranchuk

Abstract

A positive association between dilated cardiomyopathy (DCM) and Lyme disease (LD) has been shown in several small observational studies in Europe but has not been replicated in North America. In previous studies, serological testing has been a limiting factor in establishing a causal link between LD and DCM. Many trials have relied on the more accurate endomyocardial biopsy (EMB) with PCR testing of tissue. Randomized controlled trials are required to determine if there is a benefit of antibiotics in addition to standard goal-directed medial therapy in the treatment of LD-associated DCM.

Keywords

Lyme disease · Lyme carditis · Dilated cardiomyopathy · Randomized controlled trials

1 Introduction

When Lyme disease (LD) is not diagnosed or treated effectively with antibiotics during the initial weeks of infection, the bacteria *Borrelia burgdorferi* may result in manifestations of disseminated infection. In cases of early neurologic disease and

R. Wamboldt (✉) · A. Baranchuk
76 Stuart Street, Kingston, Ontario K7L 3N6, Canada
e-mail: 17reaw@queensu.ca

J. Aucott
2360 W. Joppa Road, Suite 320, Lutherville, MD 21093, US
e-mail: jaucott2@jhmi.edu

O. Cingolani
733 N Broadway, Baltimore, MD 21205, US
e-mail: ocingol1@jhmi.edu

LC, consequence of this may be seen in the first several months (Stage 2) following the original untreated infection. Late disseminated LD (Stage 3) may present clinically months or years after initial infection. It has been best documented in the skin (acrodermatitis chronica atrophicans in Europe) and in the joints (Lyme arthritis) [1].

Recently, there has been growing evidence that dilated cardiomyopathy (DCM) may be one of the late consequences of infection with LD and is covered in detail in Chap. 14 [2]. DCM is characterized by left ventricular or biventricular dilation with impaired myocardial contraction that is not explained by abnormal loading conditions such as hypertension, valvular disease, or coronary artery disease. Despite several studies showing a positive association between DCM and LD, and in some cases, improvement in cardiac function following the administration of antibiotics, research in this area has been done exclusively with small observational studies, that are underpowered and subject to confounding [2]. As such, routine testing for LD is not currently recommended in clinical guidelines for patients with idiopathic DCM [3]. There is significant potential for further research in this area to determine the true prevalence of Lyme-associated DCM and to assess whether there is a role for antibiotics in its treatment.

2 Discussion

Studies out of Europe have shown an association between *B.burgdorferi* and DCM, via endomyocardial biopsy (EMB) (tissue staining, immunohistochemistry, PCR) and serological testing, as well as improvement in cardiac function on echocardiography after antibiotic administration [4–10]. Based on these studies, the prevalence of LD amongst patients with DCM is estimated to be 20–26% [4–10]. These findings were not replicated in a single North American study, which failed to show both an association between DCM and LD or any statistically significant improvement in cardiac function on echocardiography, in a small number of patients treated with antibiotics [11]. This study however relied on clinical characteristics and serology rather than EMB used in many of the European studies. The clinical presentation, severity and virulence of LD differ between North American and European species of *B.burgdorferi* sensu lato, so it is possible that DCM is not a common manifestation of North American species [12]. Unfortunately, there is not enough data to support this hypothesis.

There are many challenges to studying LD in patients with idiopathic DCM. The accuracy of diagnostic tests in late disseminated disease remains uncertain. Early studies used ELISA testing, which has a sensitivity of around 50% in the early phases of disseminated LD and in the post-treatment phase [2, 13]. Many of the studies discussed above have included EMB specimens, which can be used to directly visualize spirochaetes and inflammation [2]. EMB in combination with western blot and qualitative serum PCR has the highest positive predictive value for *B.burgdoferi*; however EMB is an invasive procedure, not free of complications, and can be limited by sampling error [14].

Serum antibody testing is very sensitive in patients with extracutaneous manifestations, such as LC; therefore, seronegativity to immunoglobulin G (IgG) in untreated patients essentially rules out LD, if there is no humoral immunodeficient state [3]. Current guidelines from the Infectious Disease Society of America (IDSA) recommend a standard 2-tiered testing protocol (STTT), in which an enzyme immunoassay (EIA) or indirect florescent antibody test (IFA) is followed by antibody (IgM, IgG) immunoblots [3]. Alternatively, two different EIAs can be performed without the use of immunoblot testing [3]. One of the challenges with this method is that it can be difficult to determine when the initial infection occurred, as IgM and IgG for *B.burgdorferi* can persist for years after eradication of the infection [3]. Cross-reactivity can occur with antibodies to other microbes, which can also cause a false positive result [3].

Another consideration is that medial therapy for DCM has improved significantly since the publication of these observational studies on the topic of DCM and LD. Any clinical study performed to assess the benefit of antibiotics in patients with DCM and positive Lyme serology, would need to be a randomized controlled trial to determine if any measured improvement in cardiac function was secondary to the administered antibiotics or due to guideline-directed medical therapy (GDMT) alone. Additionally, there is uncertainty regarding the recommended length of antibiotics in this population. Current guidelines from the IDSA recommend ceftriaxone intravenously for 14–21 days for patients with neurologic LD and refractory Lyme arthritis [3]. Studies that have tried to treat presume Lyme-associated DCM have used a similar course of antibiotics to the IDSA guidelines with mixed results, with two studies administering intravenous ceftriaxone for 14 days and four studies administering intravenous ceftriaxone for 21 days [2]. Longer courses of antibiotics have not been shown to incur benefit and may be associated with an increased risk of side effects [15].

It is worth considering that when there is cardiac colonization, an exaggerated immune response occurs leading to cardiac injury. Animal models have shown transmural inflammation with infiltration of myocytes and lymphocytes, regardless of the presence of spirochaetes, with a predilection for perivascular regions [16]. It is possible therefore that DCM is the result of immune-mediated damage rather than ongoing active infection. In these cases, antibiotics would not be an effective treatment option for these patients.

Our lab is in the process of finalizing a research proposal to explore this association in more detail. LD is endemic in our region of southeastern Ontario and therefore, we would be able to facilitate a study with adequate power to measure an association more accurately [2]. In addition to establishing the true prevalence of Lyme-associated DCM, our study will establish whether there is any noticeable improvement in symptoms, echocardiographic parameters and MRI imaging following adequate treatment of Lyme disease in those who have highly suspected or possible Lyme-associated DCM (Fig. 1).

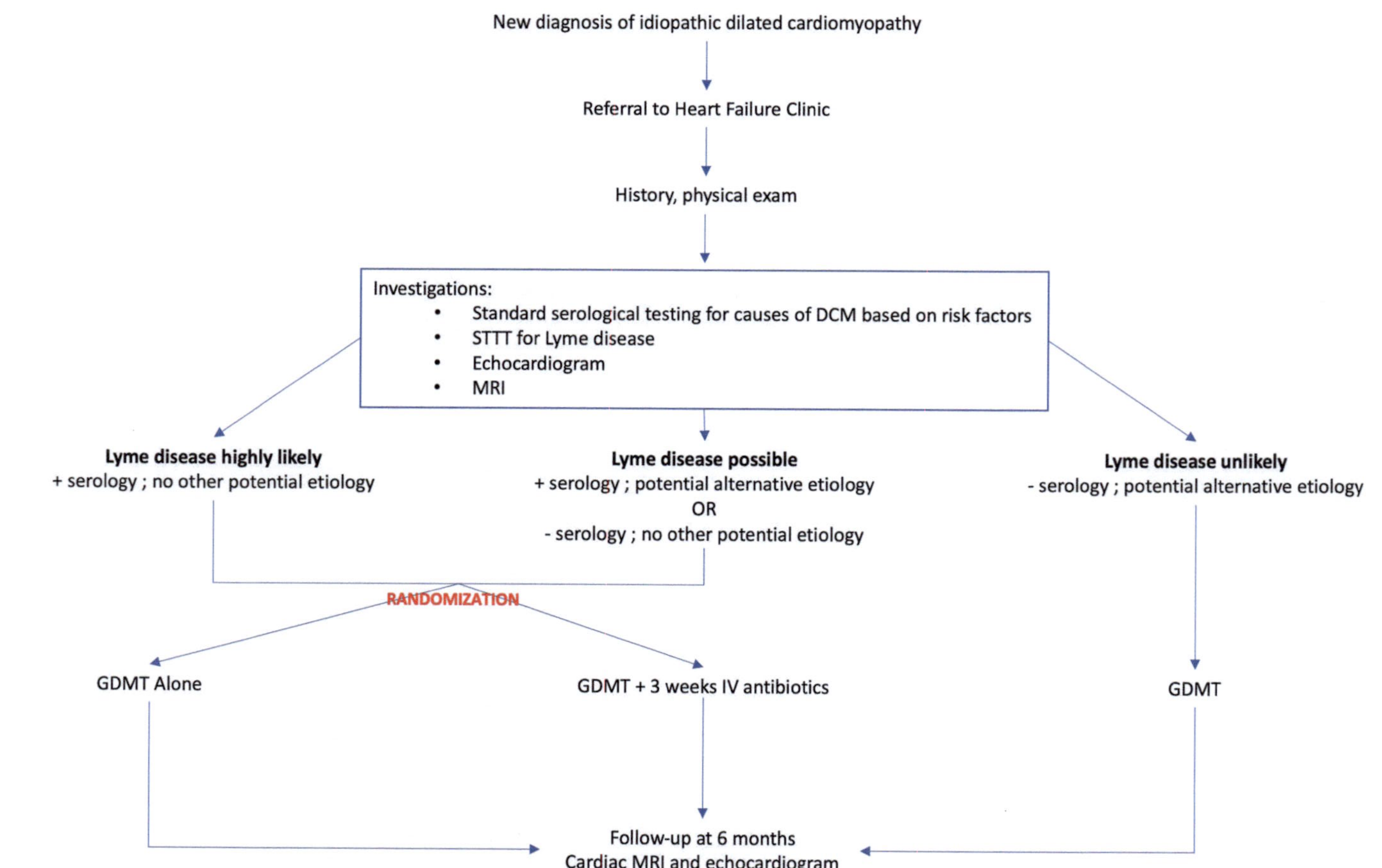

Fig. 1 Recommended RCT algorithm for patients presenting with idiopathic DCM

3 Conclusion

The true prevalence of late disseminated LD amongst those presenting with idiopathic DCM in Lyme endemic regions is likely underreported and needs to be further assessed, especially in North America. In addition, randomized controlled trials are necessary to determine whether there is a role for antibiotics in addition to standard GDMT in patients with idiopathic DCM and suspected or possible late disseminated LD.

References

1. Skar GL, Simonsen KA. Lyme disease. StatPearls [Internet]. 2022. Available from: https://www.ncbi.nlm.nih.gov/books/NBK431066/#_NBK431066_pubdet_.
2. Motamed M, Liblik K, Miranda-Arboleda AF, Wamboldt R, Wang CN, Cingolani O, Rebman AW, Novak CB, Aucott JN, Farina JM, Baranchuk A. Disseminated Lyme disease and dilated cardiomyopathy: a systematic review. Trends Cardiovascular Med. 2022; [in press] https://doi.org/10.1016/j.tcm.2022.05.010.
3. Lantos PM, Rumbaugh J, Bockenstedt LK, Falck-Ytter YT, Aguero-Rosenfeld ME, Auwaerter PG, Baldwin K, Bannuru RR, Belani KK, Bowie WR, et al. Clinical practice guidelines by the infectious diseases society of America (IDSA), American academy of neurology (AAN), and American college of rheumatology (ACR): 2020 guidelines for the prevention, diagnosis and treatment of lyme disease. Clin Infect Dis. 2021;72:e1–48.
4. Gasser R, Fruhwald F, Schumacher M, Seinost G, Reisinger E, Eber B, et al. Reversal of Borrelia burgdorferi associated dilated cardiomyopathy by antibiotic treatment? Cardiovasc Drugs Ther. 1996;10:351–60.
5. Klein J, Stanek G, Bittner R, Horvat R, Holzinger C, Glogar D. Lyme borreliosis as a cause of myocarditis and heart muscle disease. Eur Heart J. 1991;12(Suppl D):73–5.
6. Stanek G, Klein J, Bittner R, Glogar D. Borrelia burgdorferi as an etiologic agent in chronic heart failure? Scand J Infect Dis Suppl. 1991;77:85–7.
7. Karatolios K, Maisch B, Pankuweit S. Suspected inflammatory cardiomyopathy. Prevalence of Borrelia burgdorferi in endomyocardial biopsies with positive serological evidence. Herz. 2015;40 Suppl 1:91–95.
8. Bartunek P, Gorican K, Veiser T, Táborský M, Hulínská D. Significance of Bor-relia infection in development of dilated cardiomypathy (a pilot study). Prague Med Rep. 2007;108:339–47.
9. Kuchynka P, Palecek T, Havranek S, Vitkova I, Nemecek E, Trckova R, et al. Re-cent-onset dilated cardiomyopathy associated with Borrelia burgdorferi infec-tion. Herz. 2015;40:892–7.
10. Palecek T, Kuchynka P, Hulinska D, Schramlova J, Hrbackova H, Vitkova I, et al. Presence of Borrelia burgdorferi in endomyocardial biopsies in patients with new-onset unexplained dilated cardiomypathy. Med Microbiol Immunol. 2010;199:139–43.
11. Sonnesyn SW, Diehl SC, Johnson RC, Kubo SH, Goodman JL. A prospective study of the sero-prevalence of Borrelia burgdorferi infection in patients with severe heart failure. Am J Cardiol. 1995;76:97–100.
12. Yeung C, Baranchuk A. Diagnosis and treatment of lyme carditis. J Am Coll Cardiol. 2019;73(6):717–26.
13. Kubánek M, Šramko M, Berenová D, Hulínská D, Hrbáčková H, Malušková J, et al. Detection of Borrelia burgdorferi sensu lato in endomyocardial biopsy specimens in individuals with recent-onset dilated cardiomyopathy. Eur J Heart Fail. 2012;14:588–96.
14. Cooper, LT, Baughman, KL, Feldman, AM. The role of endomyocardial biopsy in the management of cardiovascular disease: a scientific statement from the American Heart Association, American College of Cardiology, and European Society of Cardiology. Endorsed by the heart

failure society of America and heart failure association of the European society of cardiology. J Am Coll Cardiol. 2007;50:1914–31.
15. Krause PJ, Bockenstedt LK. Lyme disease and the heart. Circulation. 2013;127:e451–4.
16. Cadavid D, Bai Y, Hodzic E, Narayan K, Barthold SW, Pachner AR. Cardiac involvement in non-human primates infected with the Lyme disease spirochete Borrelia burgdorferi. Lab Investig. 2004;84:1439–50.

Into the Future: New Investigations on Autoimmune Reactions Against Cardiac Structures

Penny McCreath, Adrian Baranchuk, Animesh Sinha, Meena Fatah, Diptendu Chatterjee, and Robert Hamilton

Abstract

The incidence of Lyme carditis is expected to increase due to human migration, reforestation, and climate mediated improvement. Autoantibody biomarkers of Lyme carditis can: (a) stratify affected individuals based on their risk of a sustained immune response and cardiac involvement, thereby facilitating proactive treatment regimens; and (b) be targeted in future precision medicine therapies, improving the quality of care for patients with Lyme carditis. A unique autoantibody profile of abnormally expressed cardiac proteins is likely present in Lyme disease. Discovery of biomarkers of cardiac involvement in Lyme disease will help to elucidate the sequelae leading to sustained humoral autoimmunity following initial infection with Lyme disease.

Keywords

Lyme disease • Lyme carditis • Autoantibody biomarkers • Autoantibody • Biomarkers • Autoimmunity

P. McCreath (✉) · A. Baranchuk
Division of Cardiology, Queen's University, Kingston, Canada
e-mail: penelope.mccreath@queensu.ca

A. Baranchuk
e-mail: Adrian.Baranchuk@kingstonhsc.ca

P. McCreath · M. Fatah · D. Chatterjee · R. Hamilton
Division of Cardiology, Translational Medicine, The Hospital for Sick Children, Toronto, Canada
e-mail: robert.hamilton@sickkids.ca

A. Sinha
Division of Dermatology, Immunology, University of Buffalo, Buffalo, USA
e-mail: aasinha@buffalo.edu

1 Introduction

Lyme disease (LD) is a common, vector-borne infection transmitted through the bite of infected ticks with the spirochete *Borrelia burgdoferi (B. burgdoferi)*. In the early disseminated phase, the spirochete spreads into many organ systems, which can lead to Lyme carditis (LC) if the cardiac system becomes involved [1]. The differential diagnosis of LC is complex and multi-faceted due to non-specific and heterogenous clinical manifestations [1]. Symptoms may be transient, but can also include dyspnea, palpitations, chest pain, or arrhythmic syncope [1]. LC most commonly presents as atrioventricular block (AVB), in up to 90% of cases, but can manifest as a variety of conduction and inflammatory cardiac disorders [1–3].

2 Immunopathogenesis of Lyme Carditis

The exact mechanism leading to LC is not well understood. It is hypothesized to be exacerbated by autoimmune inflammatory responses to spirochetes present in heart tissue, causing the abnormalities which can induce AV block [1]. *B. burgdoferi* (and other spirochetes) are thought to target cardiac tissue in LC by modulating the expression of its surface proteins in order to bind to the extracellular matrix, vasculature, and host tissue cells (myocardial tissue). Specifically, borrelial surface proteins, such as P66 and decorin-binding protein, are integral to cardiac tropism in the human host [1]. Upon successful colonization, an amplified immune response occurs, beginning the progression of cardiac abnormalities that induce AV block. Cross-reactive IgM antibodies react against B. burgdoferi antigens, leading to an autoimmune response against the heart that causes additional functional abnormalities [1]. Extensive literature highlights a strong correlation between the number of spirochetes in heart tissue, myocardial inflammation, and the degree of conduction abnormalities. However, it remains unclear why conduction tissue is preferentially targeted. Details of the ethiopathogenic mechanisms of LD are discussed further in Chap. 3.

3 The Clinical Significance of a Biomarker Predicting Cardiac Manifestations in LD: Our Study Concept

We aim to identify an autoantibody biomarker that can accurately predict the development of LC in individuals diagnosed with LD. The findings of this study can be used to create a prognostic test that can expedite the diagnostic process for LC. In this context, patients will be able to obtain a definitive diagnosis and actively seek treatment in a shorter time following initial infection, reducing the risk of severe cardiac complications, such as complete AVB, myocarditis, and pacemaker implantation, and ultimately improving the quality of care for critically ill patients.

We will use our previously published 2D gel discovery platform as an unbiased method to assess all cardiac protein targets of autoantibodies, sourcing these proteins from normal human ventricular myocardium, from atrioventricular node-like pacemaker cardiomyocytes developed by collaborator *S. Protze*, and from embryonic stem cell-derived Purkinje cells [4].

Proteins in the gels will be exposed to patient and control sera, and mass spectrometry will be used to identify protein targets using PEAKs® Studio software (Bioinformatics Solutions, Inc., Waterloo, Ontario). The protein targets will be cross-correlated with protein lists of similar isoelectric point and molecular weight, and gene and protein expression databases for the cardiac tissue of interest. The confirmed proteins and their epitopes will be used to develop an ELISA for clinical use, with the goal of developing new diagnostic tools and therapeutic targets for LC.

The study will use Precision for Medicine, Inc.'s normal control sera to optimize assays on our biomarker discovery platform. We have obtained U.S. LD samples with associated phenotype information (n = 13 cardiac Lyme, 10 non-cardiac Lyme) and will perform serum exposures for the 2D gels at the University of Buffalo, with the remainder of processing and analysis performed at the Sick-Kids Research Institute. Prospective validation will be done with adult patients with definite LC and corresponding non-cardiac LD controls. Blood samples will be procured from an established cardiac serum biobank study at Queen's University in Kingston, Ontario (n = 27), and their progression of LC antibodies over time will be monitored.

4   Preliminary Results and Next Steps

The preliminary 2D gel results of LD sera have identified cardiac antibodies to proteins in three regions of interest, which are absent in control sera. The distinct groups of dots, as seen in Fig. 1, represent potential cardiac targets and have been consistent across all 5 LD serum samples. The characteristics of the antibodies to proteins in the three regions of interest (see Table 1) will be used to identify specific protein candidates, which will be further confirmed by mass spectrometry. While we hypothesize that there will be different cardiac targets in LC vs non-cardiac LD, we must complete our analysis on samples with associated phenotype information (from the U.S. Lyme Disease biobank) to support this conclusion.

5   Conclusion

Our preliminary findings are promising, suggesting that a unique cardiac autoantibody profile exists in LD, when compared to controls.

In summary, we hope to apply our findings in two contexts. Firstly, to elucidate the sequelae leading to sustained humoral autoimmunity following initial infection with LD. Secondly, to inform the development a prognostic test that can expedite the diagnostic process for LC and stratify individuals based on their risk of future cardiac involvement. This would enable healthcare professionals to

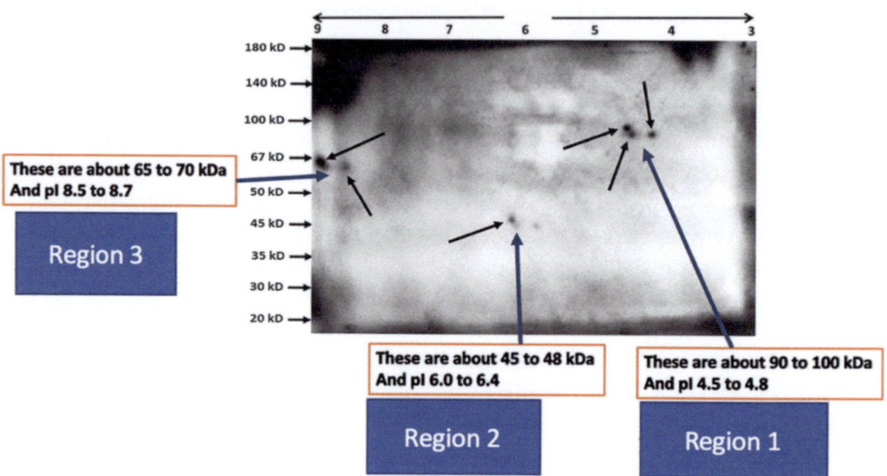

Fig. 1 Gel 2D electrophoresis with heart tissue and sera from patients with Lyme disease

Table 1 Cardiac protein candidate characteristics from Lyme disease sera

	Isoelectric point (pI)	Molecular weight (kDa)
Region 1	4.5–4.8	90–100
Region 2	6.0–6.4	45–48
Region 3	8.5–8.7	65–70

implement proactive treatment plans, ultimately serving to reduce the incidence of severe cardiac complications associated with LC.

References

1. Radesich C, Del Mestre E, Medo K, et al. Lyme carditis: from pathophysiology to clinical management. Pathogens. 2022;11(5):582. Published 2022 May 15. https://doi.org/10.3390/pathogens11050582.
2. Scheffold N, Herkommer B, Kandolf R, May AE. Lyme carditis–diagnosis, treatment and prognosis. Dtsch Arztebl Int. 2015;112(12):202–8. https://doi.org/10.3238/arztebl.2015.0202.
3. Rivera OJ, Nookala V. Lyme carditis. In: StatPearls. Treasure Island (FL): StatPearls Publishing; 2022 Feb 15.
4. Chatterjee D, et al. An autoantibody profile detects Brugada syndrome and identifies abnormally expressed myocardial proteins. Eur Heart J. 2020;41(30):2878–90.

Index

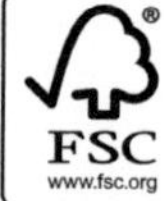